D1588079

Queen I\

ARTS THERAPIES AND THE MENTAL HEALTH OF CHILDREN AND YOUNG PEOPLE

Arts Therapies and the Mental Health of Children and Young People presents innovative international research, theory and practice in the arts therapies. The different social, cultural and political contexts and developmental age groups, illustrate and underscore the richness and diversity of contemporary arts therapies' creative response to the needs of children and young people in contrasting locations.

The book represents an acknowledgement of the high rates of mental disorders in children and young people and addresses this subject. In presenting an array of responses from arts therapists working with children and young people in different contexts and countries, the book highlights the particular features of distinct art forms, yet also points to the potential dialogue between disciplines. Chapters show how the expressive potential and appeal of the arts, when facilitated within the therapeutic relationship, are crucial in fostering hope in the future and the capacity for trust in self and others.

This book will be of great interest to arts therapists as well as academics and postgraduate students in the fields of arts therapies, social work, psychotherapy, health psychology, and education.

Uwe Herrmann is a professor on the MA Art Therapy training course at Weissensee University of Art Berlin, Germany. He has published extensively in the field of art therapy.

Margaret Hills de Zárate is an art therapist, researcher, and Honorary Senior at Queen Margaret University, Edinburgh, UK. Her publications focus on cultural issues and migration in art and art therapy.

Salvo Pitruzzella is a drama therapist and teaches arts education and dramatherapy in Italy. His many publications on these subjects include his work *Drama, Creativity, and Intersubjectivity* (Routledge, 2016).

International Research in the Arts Therapies
Series Editors: Diane Waller and Sarah Scoble

This series consists of high-level monographs identifying areas of importance across all arts therapy modalities and highlighting international developments and concerns. It presents recent research from countries across the world and contributes to the evidence-base of the arts therapies. Chapters in this series discuss and analyse current innovations and approaches in the arts therapies and arts therapies education.

This series is accessible to practitioners of the arts therapies and to colleagues in a broad range of related professions, including those in countries where arts therapies are still emerging. The monographs should also provide a valuable source of reference to government departments and health services.

Diane Waller and Sarah Scoble

Titles in the Series

1 **Intercultural Arts Therapies Research**
Issues and Methodologies
Edited by Ditty Dokter and Margaret Hills de Zárate

2 **Art Therapies and New Challenges in Psychiatry**
Edited by Karin Dannecker

3 **Arts Therapies in the Treatment of Depression**
Edited by Ania Zubala and Vicky Karkou

4 **Arts Therapies and Gender Issues**
International Perspectives on Research
Edited by Susan Hogan

5 **Arts Therapies and the Mental Health of Children and Young People**
Contemporary Research, Theory and Practice, Volume 1
Edited by Uwe Herrmann, Margaret Hills de Zárate and Salvo Pitruzzella

For more information about the series, please visit https://www.routledge.com/ International-Research-in-the-Arts-Therapies/book-series/IRAT

ARTS THERAPIES AND THE MENTAL HEALTH OF CHILDREN AND YOUNG PEOPLE

Contemporary Research, Theory, and Practice
Volume 1

Edited by Uwe Herrmann, Margaret Hills de Zárate, and Salvo Pitruzzella

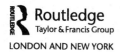
Routledge
Taylor & Francis Group

LONDON AND NEW YORK

First published 2021
by Routledge
2 Park Square, Milton Park, Abingdon, Oxon OX14 4RN

and by Routledge
605 Third Avenue, New York, NY 10158

Routledge is an imprint of the Taylor & Francis Group, an informa business

British Library Cataloguing-in-Publication Data
A catalogue record for this book is available from the British Library

Library of Congress Cataloging-in-Publication Data
A catalog record has been requested for this book

ISBN: 978-0-367-45667-2 (hbk)
ISBN: 978-1-032-01157-8 (pbk)
ISBN: 978-1-003-02466-8 (ebk)

Typeset in Bembo
by MPS Limited, Dehradun

CONTENTS

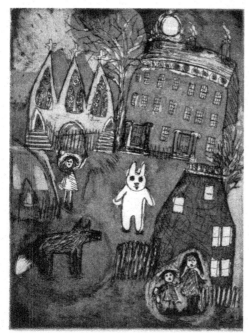

Night Rabbit– etching by Sheena McGregor 2019, Glasgow Print Studio

FIGURES

TABLES

BOXES

CONTRIBUTORS

Maika Campo completed a Bachelor of Arts in psychology at the University of the Basque Country (San Sebastian, Spain) in 2001 and a Master's degree in DMT from the Autonomous University of Barcelona (Barcelona, Spain) in 2010. She is a registered member of the Spanish DMT Association and has been employed as a Community worker since 2006. From 2011 to 2015, Maika has held DMT workshops in migration projects and has been a member of the teaching team at Masters in DMT programme at the Autonomous University of Barcelona since 2014.

Di Gammage is a dramatherapist, play therapist, Buddhist psychotherapist, child psychotherapist and accredited trainer of the Challenge of Change Resilience Training. She has contributed to the education of several generations of play therapists, dramatherapists and mindfulness-based psychotherapists in different universities and training organisations in the UK, Greece and Pakistan. She has a private practice in Devon, UK, is consultant to a private foster care agency and is a registered child psychotherapy provider to local authorities in the South West. She is author of *Playful Awakening* (2017) and has contributed a number of articles and chapters to various journals and academic books.

Tali Gottfried is a registered music therapist and a certified supervisor. She is a lecturer at the Bachelor Programme for Special Education at Herzog Academic College in Jerusalem, Israel. Tali also runs a private music therapy practice for children, adolescents and their families, and serves as the Israeli representative to the European Music Therapy Federation (EMTC). Tali has published several articles and book chapters, mostly focussed on music therapy with autistic children within a family-centred approach, and developed the Music in Everyday Life (MEL) assessment (http://mel-assessment.com).

Uwe Herrmann trained in fine art and social pedagogy in Germany, and in art psychotherapy at the University of Hertfordshire (PG Dip AT) and Goldsmiths College, University of London (Master of Research in Art Psychotherapy and PhD). In 1991, he developed the art therapy service at the State Training Institute for the Blind in Hanover, Germany, where he has continued his practice with blind and partially sighted children, adolescents and young adults to present date. Concurrently, he built up Germany's first MA programme in art therapy with Prof. Dr. Karin Dannecker at Weissensee Academy of Art Berlin, where he was appointed professor in art therapy in 2014. He has published and lectured widely on art therapy in Germany, the UK, South Korea and many countries of the European Union. His research interests are the psychodynamics of vision and congenital blindness, symbol formation, mentalization and visual/artistic methods of enquiry in art psychotherapy.

Margaret Hills de Zárate is an Honorary Senior Lecturer at Queen Margaret University in Edinburgh. Margaret trained at Goldsmith's College, Edinburgh University, the Scottish Institute of Human Relations, and the University of Havana, Cuba. She has worked and taught in various countries, including Taiwan, Spain, Argentina, Chile, Colombia, Mexico and Kenya, and latterly in Ukraine where she was curator of the Art Psychotherapy training programme affiliated to the Ukrainian Psychotherapy Association from 2010 to 2014. Her transdiciplinary research with the 'Transnationalizing Modern Languages: Mobility, Identity and Translation in Modern Italian Cultures', was funded by the UK Arts and Humanities Research Council, and is focused on material culture and our relationship with objects, and the practices and performances associated with them as a vehicle of cultural translation. Her research interests include art-based research, ethnography and migration studies.

Sheena McGregor is a graduate of Glasgow School of Art, where she studied printmaking under Philip Reeves. She was a founder member of the Glasgow Print Studio before teaching in Further Education, including nine years as art tutor in HMP Barlinnie. Seeing at first hand, the effects of childhood deprivation on addiction and social exclusion in inmates led her to train as an art therapist, graduating from Queen Margaret University in 2000. Since 2001, Sheena has worked as Lead Art Therapist for Creative Therapies, Glasgow, a charity which has developed innovative ways of using the arts to address mental health issues in children and young people. Sheena has clinical experience running art therapy groups for mothers with postnatal depression, and with fostered and adopted children. Since 2004, Sheena has worked at the Royal Hospital for Children in Glasgow, delivering art therapy in both individual and group settings for children with early onset, severe mental health difficulties in the National Child Psychiatric In-patient Unit, and also running groups for children with heart conditions.
She has lectured and presented her work at conferences and seminars in Chile, Germany, Poland, Italy and Lithuania. This has been supported by lecturing at Queen Margaret University, in the Department of Health Sciences, Nursing,

Occupational Therapy, Art and Music Therapy. She has maintained her visual art practice, running alongside her therapeutic work, producing ceramics, printmaking and painting, with work held in private and public collections.

Karen McLeod is a consultant in paediatric cardiology and electrophysiology at the Royal Hospital for Children in Glasgow. She is regularly invited to speak at local, national and international conferences on heart rhythm disorders in children and has a number of publications on the subject.

Michael Morton gained his first degree in medical science and history of art at Sidney Sussex College, Cambridge. He completed clinical training first in medicine and then in psychiatry in Edinburgh. After 18 months of further training in the NHS therapeutic community based in Dingleton Hospital, Melrose, he undertook higher specialist training in child and adolescent psychiatry in Manchester. He returned to Scotland as a consultant, working first in Dumfries and then for 18 years as a consultant child and adolescent psychiatrist in the Royal Hospital for Sick Children, Yorkhill, Glasgow. He was clinical lead during the commissioning of the National In-patient Psychiatric Unit for Children and also led the development of Liaison Psychiatry in the Children's Hospital. The experience of learning to observe both as a doctor and as an art historian informed his interest in children's communication through creative activity and in the integration of art therapy into clinical practice.

Heidrun Panhofer is the co-founder, former president and supervising member of the Spanish Association of Dance Movement Therapy (ADMTE). She has a PhD in dance movement therapy, University of Hertfordshire, and a Master's in Dance Movement Therapy, Laban Center for Movement and Dance, London City University, England. Heidrun was the editor of the compilation of the first book on dance movement therapy to be published in Spanish *The Body in Psychotherapy: Theory and Practice of Dance Movement Therapy* (2005). Heidrun is a teacher in several masters in DMT in Spain and other countries.

Salvo Pitruzzella is a pioneer of dramatherapy in Italy. Starting from a background as an actor, playwright and puppeteer, he has been working as a dramatherapist for over 25 years in different fields, mainly mental health, education and life-long, and social care. In 1998, he founded the first dramatherapy training course in Italy at the 'Centro ArtiTerapie', Lecco of which he is still a teacher and scientific advisor. Since 2012, he has lectured in arts education and creative writing at the Fine Arts Academies of Palermo and Bari, Italy. He is international member of the BADTh (British Association of Dramatherapists), and member of the Editorial Advisory Board of *Dramatherapy Journal*. He is Honorary Member of SPID (Società Professionale Italiana di Drammaterapia), on behalf of which he attends the Executive Board of the EFD (European Federation of Dramatherapy), which includes the professional associations of seventeen European countries. Moreover, he is Italian Regional Representative at ECArTE (European Consortium for Arts Therapies Education). Since 2013, he has been co-editor of the ECArTE publications (with Malcolm Ross,

Sarah Scoble, Richard Hougham and Hilda Wengrower). He has lectured and led workshops all around Italy, as well as in the UK, Israel, Switzerland, Malta, Romania, Czech Republic, Greece, Belgium, the USA, Malta, Germany and Poland.

He has widely published on dramatherapy, educational theatre and creativity theories, including the recent *Drama, Creativity and Intersubjectivity: Foundations of Change in Dramatherapy*, London, Routledge, 2016.

Rosemarie Samaritter is a licensed senior dance movement therapist and supervisor. Her work is rooted in her studies in Dalcroze rhythmics, modern dance, dance movement therapy, integrative movement therapy and short-term experiential dynamic therapy.

She has extensive clinical experience in outpatient settings in the Dutch National Health Services and in private practice with children, adolescents and adults. She has specialised in dyadic DMT intervention in personality disorders, trauma and psychopathologies related to a disturbed sense of self and attachment trauma. Rosemarie was involved in the development of the first professional DMT programmes in the Netherlands. She has been teaching DMT theory and methodology in various DMT programmes in the Netherlands and abroad. She has been involved in the Dutch national licensing procedures of new training programmes for creative arts therapies and works as DMT representative on the development of national guidelines. Currently she works as a programme research leader and supervisor on the Master of Arts Therapies Education at Codarts Rotterdam (NL). As a researcher, she is involved in intervention research and the development of innovative DMT research projects with a specific focus on dance-informed research strategies.

Sarah Soo Hon is a registered art therapist and doctoral student at Queen Margaret University, Edinburgh. She facilitates individual and group art therapy in inpatient, outpatient and forensic settings in the North West Regional Health Authority in Trinidad and Tobago. She serves as public relations officer of the Autistic Society of Trinidad and Tobago and is a founding member of the Art Therapy Association of Trinidad and Tobago. Her current area of research seeks to understand the relevance of cultural art practices to the psychosocial wellbeing of adolescents affected by violence in Trinidad and Tobago.

Daniel Stolfi is a UK-based dramatherapist, medical anthropologist and the artistic director of The Awesome Puppet Company. He is a core tutor and academic support lead for the MA programme in child and adolescent psychotherapy at Terapia in London as well as the organization's institutional link tutor with Middlesex University. He has been a visiting lecturer at the Royal Central School of Speech & Drama and Anglia Ruskin University in the UK and has also presented his work extensively in the USA, including NYU Steinhardt and the California Institute of Integral Studies (CIIS). He has a specialist interest in the therapeutic uses of puppetry, and how our understanding and experience of suffering and healing are informed by, and reproduce social and cultural value. He is active in education, training, research and publishing in these fields.

Heike Wrogemann-Becker is a government-licensed music pedagogue and a certificated music therapist. She studied musical education at Musikhochschule Lübeck, Music- and Movement Pedagogy (Teaching diploma) at Mozarteum (Orff-Institut) Salzburg (Austria), Music Therapy (Diploma) at Hochschule für Musik und Theater Hamburg. Heike was awarded a Ph.D. by Hochschule für Musik und Theater Hamburg with a dissertation on how music therapy can enhance the symbol formation of congenitally blind children. After extended practice in child and youth education, she has been working in music therapy with children, adolescents and adults over the past 15 years. Heike has taught on the special education teacher-training course at Musikhochschule Hamburg and has also been working as a music therapist at a psychosomatic clinic in Germany for the past eight years.

THE ARTS THERAPIES AND THE MENTAL HEALTH IN CHILDREN AND YOUNG PEOPLE: AN INTRODUCTION

Margaret Hills de Zárate and Uwe Herrmann

In 1995, Nelson Mandela was to state that 'there is no keener revelation of a society's soul than the way in which it treats its children' (Mandela, 1995). A quarter of a century later, a report published by the WHO–UNICEF–Lancet Commission (Clark et al., 2020) reveals that the social, physical and psychological health of children and young people is more at risk than ever. Yet as this report concludes, the evidence is clear: 'early investments in children's health, education, and development have benefits that compound throughout the child's lifetime, for their future children, and society as a whole' (Clark et al., p. 605).

This book is the first of several collections of papers which address the mental health of children and young people in the ECArTE/ICRA series International Research in the Arts Therapies. This first volume presents nine chapters from eight countries (England, Germany, Italy, Trinidad Tobago, Spain, Scotland, Israel and the Netherlands). These distinct contexts, along with their specific historical, political, cultural and social factors, have informed mental health policies and mental health care provision for children and young people and influenced the practice of arts therapists.

The mental health of children and young people: new challenges

As distinct as these chapters are, in terms of historic background, social conditions and geographical location, they reveal a picture, incomplete but indicative, of the lives of children and young people in the wider context of globalisation. A ubiquitous term, globalisation tries to capture the rapid social change that is occurring simultaneously across a multiplicity of dimensions. This includes the economic, political and the social, which in turn encompass the interpersonal, informational and cultural (Dey, 2017; Gygli et al., 2019) Globalisation impacts upon the contexts and the lives of the young people with whom arts therapists work and particularly those who are already disadvantaged by the glaring inequalities which 'we see all the time, whether at the school gates, the hospital, when travelling round the country – or even a single town – or when turning on the news' (The IFS Deaton Review, 2020).

The examples of contemporary arts therapies theory, practice and research presented in this first collection of chapters reflect the current landscape of engagement with children and young people; however, even in the richest countries the key underlying issues remain, namely social inequality, child poverty and deprivation.[1] In recent years, there have been very interesting developments in art therapy practice, for example in the area of mentalization, and yet some of the fundamental theoretical ideas, those of the unconscious, sublimation and symbolisation which informed the development of arts therapies maintain their currency as does the centrality of the specific art form. One example from art therapy is the Austrian-American art therapy pioneer Edith Kramer, who was very clear that in art therapy, art is the main therapeutic agent, while the therapist's understanding of art is informed by their own artistic proficiency, but equally by the insights provided by psychoanalysis. However, Kramer also stressed that art, and hence art therapy, was not only about the workings of the individual psyche, but inseparable from the social, economic and political context in which each individual is embedded (Kramer, 1958, 1971, 1979). In Kramer's first book, and one of the first key texts ever written on art therapy, she presents her work in an institution for young homeless boys in New York. Here, she pinpoints the connection between poverty, implicit racism and children's mental health and advocated the use of the arts as a royal road to restore a child's mental and physical wellbeing.

Kramer (1958) made an acerbic diagnosis of a school system that failed to accommodate children from poor and underprivileged families.

> The child who is burdened with conflict and frustration in the family and harassed by the necessity for vigilant self-defence on the street, has little energy left for learning and for growth … Failure at school usually means failure at learning to read, and, if the child does not acquire this basic technique most other avenues of academic learning remain closed to him. The child then never experiences the widening of horizons and the elation of an increasing understanding and mastery of the world which should be the great experience of childhood. School and learning, which can become a steadying and healing factor in a disturbed child's life can become instead another source of conflict and bitterness.
>
> *(Kramer 1958, pp.30–31)*

In her later books, Kramer also stressed how the material assets of an increasingly consumerist society were in fact hampering children's creativity and left them, though 'materially rich' emotionally depleted (1971, 1979). Reading Kramer's work, one thing comes through very clearly throughout her writing: her strong conviction, supported by an abundance of case-based evidence, that art therapy, and the arts themselves, were a life saver for children who were otherwise lost to, and excluded from, the cultural riches of society. The arts, she argues, allow for self-expression, the building of sound ego structures, the forming of relationships, and can instil a sense of worth, belonging and being seen in children who had all but lost hope.

Looking at the array of concerns presented in this present book reveals that while parts of our societies have grown materially richer, and other parts of our societies have become more impoverished and segregated, children's lives have become less secure and less emotionally fulfilling. The same troubles that Kramer met in her work in New York from the 1950s to the early 1980s still trouble children's lives today. This is an alarming observation that does not only derive from the personal experiences of the editors and contributors to this book but is based on hard facts as laid out by the World Health Organization (WHO).

The World Health Organization Mental Health Atlas (2014a) estimates that worldwide 10–20% of children and adolescents experience mental disorders. Evidence suggests that antecedents of adult mental disorders can be detected in children and adolescents (Malhotra and Sahoo, 2018) while Kessler et al., (2007) report that half of all lifetime cases of mental disorders start by age 14 with anxiety and personality disorders sometimes beginning around the age of 11 (OECD, 2018).[2] Neuropsychiatric conditions are the leading cause of disability in young people in all regions which if untreated, severely influence children's development, their educational attainments and their potential to live fulfilling and productive lives. Amongst the most vulnerable children are those with a learning disability, autism, looked after and adopted children and those children with physical conditions such as cancer, heart conditions, epilepsy and diabetes and those affected by the impact of child poverty (WHO, 2014a). On average across OECD countries, 13.1% of children live in relative income poverty but rates differ considerably from country to country. Of these, in Chile, Israel, Spain and Turkey, more than 20% of children live in relative poverty while rates are particularly high, at around 25%, in Israel and Turkey (OECD, 2019).

In the United States, a high-income country, children remain the poorest age group. Nearly 1 in 6 children lived in poverty in 2018, that is, a total of 11.9 million children. The child poverty rate (16%) is nearly one-and-a-half times higher than that for adults (11%) and two times higher for adults of 65 years and older (10%). Child poverty is related to both age and race/ethnicity and nearly 73% of poor children in America are children of colour. Nearly 1 in 3 are Black and American Indian/Alaska Native children and 1 in 4 Hispanic children, compared with 1 in 11 of white children. The youngest children under six years are the poorest group, half of which lived in extreme poverty, 50% below the poverty line. In 2017, the Black infant mortality rate was more than two times that of White and Hispanic infants (The Children's Defense Fund, 2020 p.48), while worldwide the average risk of dying remains twice as high for children born in the poorest households compared to the richest under-five mortality rate by wealth quintile in low- and middle-income countries for the period 1990–2018 (UNICEF, 2019a, p.19).

UNICEF reports alarmingly high rates of self-harm, suicide and anxiety among children and young people around the world. According to the latest data up to 20% of adolescents globally experience mental disorders. The cost of poor mental health goes beyond the individual and the personal and has societal and economic repercussions and yet, child and adolescent mental health has often been over-looked in global and national health programming.

The reports issued by the WHO and UNICEF confirm what we, as practising arts therapists and researchers already know from a grass roots level, and it leaves us with a deep sense of crisis. There is a multitude of problems that do not only overshadow but often destroy the lives of children and young people before they have even begun.

Socio-economic conditions impact the way that parents relate to and bring up their children; thus, the increasing and pervasive economic pressures on the majority of our populations take a massive toll on those who will constitute our future societies. We are confronted with disturbing statistics on child and adolescent poverty, racism The Children's Defense Fund 2020, Trent 2019, lack of training and employment, a rise in child suicide, childhood deprivation and social exclusion (The Children's Defense Fund, 2020; Trent et al., 2019). But even in economically affluent communities, childhood seems to be changing rapidly into an odd system of highly controlled activities on the one hand, indicating a fear of non-structured play and activities, and an uncontrolled and lonely parallel world governed by digital and virtual gadgets on the other hand (OECD, 2019). Both phenomena are highly detrimental to creativity and thus to those functions in each individual psyche – and communities – that could help to build the resilience that children and young people need to master the difficult task of growing up.

The rapid digital developments in particular are raising questions as to how detrimental they are to the mental health and wellbeing of children and young people. Recent surveys and reports from the UK note that there is a strong association between high rate social media use and mental and emotional disorders in children and young people, though the exact workings remain unclear (NHS, 2018; House of Commons Science and Technology Committee, 2019). However, research suggests that digital media use interferes with parent–child interaction on a large scale, and that *parents'* problematic use of such media seriously undermines their vital, early relationship forming with their children (McDaniel and Radesky, 2017; Globokar, 2018). As traditional skills and crafts have largely disappeared from the vocational field in many societies, the arts are in a crucial position as fields of experience where individual and collective creativity can be learned and developed.

A number of chapters in this volume present research, while others offer examples of innovative practice that has matured enough to be at a point where research is called for or imminent. Not all research undertaken in the arts therapies is of a kind that sits easily with the medical model and its main paradigm of evidence-based inquiry. This is to do with the nature of the arts and the kind of processes that we instigate in the service of healing, where sometimes what is defined as Evidence-Based Practice (EBP) may or may not be a useful to examine the effects that the arts have on patients' lives. However, the arts and the arts therapies have a strong ally in the WHO and the Health Evidence Network (HEN) synthesis report on arts and health, charting the global academic literature, looking at over 900 publications, including 200 reviews that covered over 3000 further studies (WHO, 2019a). This most comprehensive and current report, evaluating existing research and practice, found strong evidence for the arts' playing a crucial, efficient and cost-effective part in the mental health and wellbeing of people in relation to an abundance of conditions. The report found evidence of the arts therapies' efficacy in the prevention of illness and promotion of health, in seveal ways: advancing social cohesion and diminishing social inequalities; enhancing child development and mother–child interaction and bonding; supporting the acquisition of speech and language; or in effectively helping socially excluded and neglected children and young people who cannot be reached in any other way. On the side of management and treatment, the report stresses the important role of the arts and the arts therapies in treating mental illnesstrauma and abuse, in acute conditions, neurological disorders, the psycho-social impact of physical illnesses, and in supporting people in palliative care and bereavement (WHO, 2019a).

In the face of these developments, it is inevitable that many subjects must be left untouched in this book, or surface only in passing, for example, child poverty, gender identity, bullying, migration, children seeking asylum and racism. Around 15% of adolescents in lowand middle-income countries have considered suicide; alarmingly, suicide is the third leading cause of death among 15–19-year-olds worldwide (UNICEF, 2019b) and one of the top-five causes of death among children aged 10–14 years in many countries in the European region in 2016 (Kyu et al., 2018). While depression remains one of the leading causes of illness and disability among adolescents (WHO, 2014a, 2019c), computer and gaming addiction appeared in the 11th revision of the International Classification of Diseases (ICD-11) in June 2018 (OECD, 2018; WHO, ICD 11, 2018).

Children and adolescents with learning disabilities are over six times more likely to have a diagnosable psychiatric disorder than their peers who do not have learning disabilities (Bond/Young Minds, 2014, p.5) and potentially a conservative estimate, given that symptoms of poor mental health in young people with disabilities are often misattributed as inherent to the disability and mental illness in this group is commonly under-diagnosed (Austin et al., 2018).

All these are pressing issues to be addressed in further volumes on the arts therapies and the mental health of children and young people. This book does, however, assemble a number of positions from practice to research that tackle vital issues that have been equally stressed by the recent WHO report on the role of the arts in promoting health and wellbeing (WHO, 2019a). In this sense, there could not be a better moment for its publication.

Contemporary arts therapies responses: chapter synopses

The following papers will exemplify why the arts therapies are fundamental agents for change, connectivity and healing for the increasing numbers of those children who are left with little or no hope for a life that could be safe and fulfilling. To them, the arts therapies have been a game changer, as the ensuing chapters will show.

Children can benefit from the arts therapies in a wide range of institutional and organisational contexts. Schools are certainly one of the areas where children with different needs and diverse backgrounds stay for extended periods of time. It is here that the arts therapies can show their potential as short- and long-term interventions. However, far from being an easy and continuous flow in which relationships are allowed to persist and mature, school time is marked by phases and transitions that can be difficult for the child to cope with. The book therefore opens with a first chapter by Di Gammage from England/UK on play psychotherapy. Children's play contains the seeds of all the art forms, and, due to its fluidity from structured to unstructured, lends itself easily to children's varying mental and physical needs.

Gammage investigates the question how play psychotherapy can help pupils in their sixth year to build resilience for their transition into secondary school. Particularly children with a pre-existing diagnosis of anxiety and depression are vulnerable to such transitions as they undo their relationships to peers, teachers and environments and transfer them to the unfamiliar. Gammage presents an action-based pilot study, aimed at determining children's levels of resilience before and after a 20session play psychotherapy programme. Using a questionnaire built on established empirical knowledge, eight key factors were scrutinised that enhance or hamper emotional resilience in the children. Gammage particularly stresses how play psychotherapy strengthens the children's mindfulness and emotional resilience. She also shows how research can constitute, and inform, live practice and can offer a promising path forward. Her work adds an important and novel building block to an educational practice where the children's psychological needs and development are not seen as an impediment, but rather *central* to their learning progress.

To thrive and develop children must establish relationships in many directions: parents, siblings, peers and teachers, to name a few. As Gammage has shown, play psychotherapy can help children with pre-existing problems to cope with being exposed to the uncertain and the unfamiliar.

In chapter 2, Tali Gottfried from Israel looks at a group of children where the uncertain and the unfamiliar are built into the core child–parent relationship from the very beginning: children with autistic spectrum disorder and their neurotypical parents must learn to understand each other and communicate by bridging the gap between their different neurological dispositions. This ongoing experience can be, at times, alienating, frustrating and challenging for both parents and children, and it is here that Gottfried offers a well-crafted and dovetailed model of music therapy that includes parent counselling alongside individual music therapy for their children. This ecological model is innovative, because it addresses the entire system of relationships rather than just the individual child and because it uses music therapy techniques in parent counselling rather than verbal exchange only.

Gottfried thus shows how an evidence-based clinical model can reduce the level of parental stress and enrich the quality of life for the parents' and the entire family by providing parents with a hands-on experience of how to use music in relating to, and communicating with, their children with autism.

In chapter 3, Daniel Stolfi from the UK/South Africa explores the role and uses of puppetry and puppet-craft in clinical dramatherapy practice with children and adolescents. Stolfi observes that puppetry, and especially puppet-craft, yet awaits systematic scrutiny and stringent theorisation to show its full potential for the clinical field. To fill this gap, he takes us along some of the less explored straits of thinking and contextualises the modality within diverse cultural and symbolic practices. Stolfi draws on his expertise from dramatherapy, medical anthropology and puppetry to provide us with a rich theoretical background for practice and research in relation to the puppet object in dramatherapy. Highlighting the qualities inherent to the actual making of the puppet-object, Stolfi theorises the puppet's intersubjective and interobjective dynamics grounded in its spatial and material dimensions. These dynamics allow the puppet to take on its role as a transformative and integrative agent that serves the relationship between self and other. Stolfi argues for a therapeutic practice that is firmly arts-based in favour of models that, for their empirical or medical framework, fail to grasp the aesthetic and symbolic complexities inherent to the arts therapies. His chapter thus shows that the arts therapies, in theory and practice, are essentially interlinked by their mutual use of, and concern with, the question of artistic form in relation to the mind and spirit of its maker.

In chapter 4, Rosemarie Samaritter from the Netherlands presents a research-based model of dance movement therapy (DMT) for children and adolescents. Considering DMT concepts combined with conclusions from neuropsychology and developmental psychology, she offers a developmental aesthetic perspective on DMT as treatment and support. As current investigations have revealed, even before a child is born the rhythms and tension of the shared maternal body strongly impact the child's physical and relational development. As this prenatal influence continues in later life, DMT is shown as a therapeutic agent that can uniquely engage children in non-verbal intersubjective exchange and address their sensor-imotor organisation within movement experiences that are, or become, symbolic.

Providing case material from clinical practice, Samaritter illustrates the shared corporal practice that is inherent to DMT and its rhythmic, expressive and aes-thetic structures. She also stresses that dance, as socio-cultural activity and as a shared aesthetic experience, can mutually enrich the dancers' social environment and enhance the children's socio-emotional integration.

Among the most precarious factors endangering the mental and physical health of children and young people are failed attachment, traumatic experiences and violence.

The psychosocial wellbeing of children and young people is highly endangered in thosewho experience violence in their families, schools and wider communities , especially in societies which are already struggling with racial and economic inequality and colonial histories.

Adolescence is one of the most rapid phases of human development. However, the timing and the speed of change varies and is influenced by both individual and external factors. Some adolescents are at greater risk due to their living conditions, stigma, discrimination, exclusion, or lack of access to quality support and services. Despite these setbacks, there is a significant window of opportunity in adolescence. We now know that the adolescent brain has significant neural plasticity, that is, it is still able to change and there is the potential in adolescence to ameliorate the impact of negative experiences earlier in life (WHO, 2014b; UNICEF, 2017).

These issues are reflected in chapter 5, by Sarah Soo Hon from Trinidad and Tobago who explores the use of artistic and musical practices for adolescents who have experienced violence in their families, communities and schools. Using a participatory ethnographic approach and encouraging adolescents to collaborate in the research, Soo Hon shows how story-telling, graffiti, song and performance provides adolescents with a voice to express and share their feelings of sadness, grief and loss. The arts, Soo Hon argues, help participants to strike the balance between their needs as individuals and their roles as part of a collective; given the unspeakable nature of being exposed to violence or being an active part in it, the arts served as a crucial agent that could moderate the adolescents' conflicting needs to retain privacy and to make a public statement about their hard-to-voice experiences.

In chapter 6, Maika Campo and Heidrun Panhofer from Spain explore how a dance movement therapist worked with failed attachment and traumatic experiences in juvenile offenders. Presenting a case study of an adolescent boy, they ground their practice firmly in attachment theory and demonstrate how the boy gradually grew to use dance and movement to tell his story, clarify his family and ethnic background and gain a new and more stable perspective on his life, past, present and future. Campo and Panhofer scrutinise how working with the body opened an avenue for reconstructing safe attachment; in this process, dance, play and movement functioned as the main agents that could offer an intercorporeal relationship providing a young person with a unique access to his early developmental stages. Through this work, the boy could confront and heal his traumatic experiences that were stored in his trauma body memory. The authors attribute the efficacy of this work to a shared corporeity serving as a tool to overcome trauma and loss. This study shows that the grim reality facing young offenders, and their perspective on their future life, can be changed by something which is as simple and inexpensive as it is complex and priceless: a form of art that can be created on the spot by and with the means of the body from virtually nothing. Of equal importance was the presence of a witnessing, appreciating dance movement therapist who was able to engage a young person to move together in shared space.

In Chapter 7 Heike Wrogemann-Becker from Germany considers children with sensory and cognitive disabilities who are at a particular risk of developmental delays and mental disorders. The ways these distinct areas are connected are often difficult to untangle. Wrogemann-Becker presents her research on individual music therapy with a cohort of six congenitally blind children and describes how music therapy enhanced the children's delayed ego-development and communicative abilities. She found that the children's ability to symbolise through music developed in distinct phases. Alongside, the specific relationship between the blind child and the sighted music therapist took on an increasingly intersubjective note. This is particularly noteworthy as Wrogemann-Becker describes how the growth of the child's symbolising functions is engendered by the child–adult relationship, which, at the same time, is hampered by the sensory gap that divides them. Consequently, she addresses the usefulness of her music therapy interventions in this process and outlines further areas of research from which blind children and their families might benefit in future. One of these unexplored areas, Wrogemann-Becker concludes, is meeting the need of the parents for someone to mediate and explain their blind children's behaviour and inner world to them so they can truly engage with their children. Wrogemann-Becker's call for future research and possibly for integrated music therapy practice dovetails with Gottfried's model of music oriented counselling for the parents of autistic children in chapter 2. Both authors thus draw on evidence from practice and research and build a strong argument for the role of music therapy for children who are different. By approaching from opposite ends – blind children's individual development towards symbolisation (Wrogemann-Becker) and making music therapy available to parents (Gottfried) – both chapters propose viable means to close the gap created by the sensory or neurological divergence between these children and their parents.

In chapter 8, Salvo Pitruzzella from Italy describes dramatherapy with adolescents in a day centre for young people with personality disorders. Scrutinising the notions of the emerging self in adolescence from the perspectives of psychology and the neurosciences, he takes us through the changes and fragmentations of this remarkable and perilous developmental phase. In this period, and particularly for young people with personality disorders, Pitruzzella suggests, the arts therapies are decisive due to their symbolic, creative, flexible and relationship-based properties. Presenting his case-based research on dramatherapy with this group, Pitruzzella grounds his practice and research on the hypothesis of the dramatic self and identifies its four essential components – narratives, roles, relationships and knowledge –through which the dramatic reality of the stage emerges in theatre and dramatherapy, and which constitute the dramatic interface system between the individual person and the world. Pitruzzella exemplifies his thoughts through a case study on dramatherapy with an adolescent girl; here he shows how the hypothesis of the dramatic self, and its four key components, surfaced in the therapeutic process and leads to a remarkable change in the girl's view of herself and her interactions with the group. Such change, he concludes, fostered within an empathetic and creative environment, demonstrates the flexible and multifaceted potential of theatre for helping the adolescent mind to master this difficult phase in life.

In chapter 9, Sheena McGregor (Art Therapy), Dr Karen McLeod (cardiology) and Dr Michael Morton (liaison psychiatry) from Scotland, UK, describe how the collaboration between three disciplines – art therapy, psychiatry and cardiac nursing – leads to innovative practice for children with chronic heart diseases. The psychological needs of these children are inseparable from their physical ones and yet have often been neglected over the severe implications of their medical problems. The collaboration of these professionals was sparked off by the case of one girl with a cardiac condition, who used art therapy in a very effective way. This inspired further thought in the team and eventually led to the instigation of a novel Cardiac Art Therapy Clinic from which a multitude of children have been able to benefit since. This chapter exemplifies how a single therapeutic initiative, focused on a particular individual, leads to a new, much needed and lasting service provision, which, in turn, generated questions and ideas that prepare the ground for future research. The authors exemplify to all of the arts therapies and in a fresh, hopeful and inspiring way that one initiative from dedicated, diverse professionals, can chart new territory and change the quality of life for children and young people with complex needs and conditions.

Conclusion and outlook

In summary, this collection of chapters shows that the arts, due to their flexible, multifaceted and creative nature, are strong allies in attempts to support and improve children's lives. In the arts therapies, we suggest that it is the doing and the making aspects of our respective artistic disciplines that makes a deep and decisive initial impression on our young clients, enables them to risk committing to the therapeutic relationship and "to stay the course" in therapy. Artists, when entering the artistic process, delve into the unknown, learn to make changes to the performance or the artwork, are equally and simultaneously changed by their work, and while in the process, learn to hold on to the hope that in the end, their efforts will lead to a good-enough resolution.

In our view, the arts therapies are ideally suited to optimise resilience in children and young people and fulfil the criteria that research has identified predisposes children to positive outcomes in the face of significant adversity. These are facilitating supportive adult–child relationships; building a sense of self-efficacy and perceived control; providing opportunities to strengthen adaptive skills and self-regulatory capacities; and mobilising sources of faith, hope and cultural traditions (National Scientific Council on the Developing Child, 2015).

Even when young clients' trust in human relationships is highly compromised, engaging in the creative process within the context of the therapeutic relationship may lead to a way forward to discover and trust in their own inherent creativity, as evidenced in the chapters to follow.

Many issues and fields of practice remain to be explored in future volumes on the mental health of children and young people. As arts therapies services are springing up rapidly in many parts of our globalised world, a much more varied picture emerges of our approaches to practice and theory, modifying and adding to the perspectives developed in the UK, the United States and the EU over the past decades. In future volumes of the ECArTE/ICRA series, on the mental health of children and young people, local socio-political contexts and cultural traditions of such new arts therapies services will continue to offer as much food for thought as their varied clientele and their needs. Such considerations, however, have long stopped being tied to geography. Global mobility and migration are likely to accelerate, urging an unprecedented cultural sensitivity and knowledge in each professional, university teacher and policy maker. This series will therefore continue to invite and present new perspectives from the many and distinct countries and contexts in Asia, Africa and South America alongside novel approaches and developments in the EU, the chapter 2 UK and the United States in subsequent volumes 2 and 3.

It is the editors' hope that such new outlooks, evidencing the varied developments in our fields, will induce change in the reader's understanding of the issues at stake and of the practices and paradigms employed to improve the mental life of children and young people. We believe that paying close attention to the intricacies of the arts, with their unparalleled flexibility, mutability and adaptivity, holds the key to an increasingly global, varied and refined understanding of our developing professions and services.

Notes

1 See: UNICEF 2017, Building the Future Children and the Sustainable Development Goals in Rich Countries.
2 The Organisation for Economic Co-operation and Development is an intergovernmental economic organisation with 37 member countries, founded in 1961 to stimulate economic progress and world trade.

References

Austin, K.L. et al. (2018) 'Depression and anxiety symptoms during the transition to early adulthood for people with intellectual disabilities', *Journal of Intellectual Disability Research*, 62(5), pp. 407–421.

Bennett, A. and Robards, B. (2014) 'Youth, cultural practice and media technologies' in Bennett, A. et al. (eds.) *Mediated youth cultures*. London: Palgrave Macmillan.

Bond/Young Minds (2014) *Children and young people with learning disabilities – Understanding their mental health* [Online]. Available at: https://www.mentalhealth.org.uk/publications/children-and-young-people-learning-disabilities-and-their-mental-health (Accessed: 1 July 2020).

Centre for Suicide Prevention (2013) *Not a child, children and suicide resource toolkit* [Online]. https://www.suicideinfo.ca/wp-content/uploads/2016/08/Childrens-Toolkit_Print.pdf (Accessed: 30 June 2020).

The Children's Defense Fund (2020) The state of America's children – 2020, Child Poverty, Children's Defense Fund [Online]. Available at: https://www.childrensdefense.org/content/uploads/2020/02/the-state-of-americas-children-2020.pdf (Accessed: 21 January 2021).

Clark, H. et al. (2020) 'A future for the world's children? A WHO–UNICEF–Lancet Commission', Lancet Commissions, 395(10224), May 21, pp. 605–658.

Dey, M. (July 2017) 'Impact of globalisation on childhood: A case study of the children of a suburban area', International Journal of Social Science Research, 7(7), pp. 567–577.

Faas, S. et al., (2019) 'Globalization, transformation, and cultures: Theoretical notes and perspectives on reconceptualization and international comparison in early childhood Education and care' in Faas, S., Kasüschke, D., Nitecki, E., Urban, M., and Wasmuth, H. (eds), Globalization, transformation, and cultures in early childhood education and care. Critical cultural studies of childhood. London: Palgrave Macmillan. 1–14.

Globokar, R. (2018) 'Impact of digital media on emotional, social and moral development of children', Nova prisutnost, 16(3), pp. 545–560 [Online]. Available at: https://doi.org/10.31192/np.16.3.8 (Accessed: 5 September 2019).

Gygli, S. et al. (2019) 'The KOF Globalisation Index – Revisited', Review of International Organizations, 2019(14), pp. 543–574. [Online]. Available at: https://doi.org/10.1007/s11558-019-09344-2 (Accessed: 9 July 2020).

House of Commons Science and Technology Committee (2019)'Impact of social media and screen-use on young people's health', Fourteenth Report of Session 2017–19 Report, together with formal minutes relating to the report, Published on 31 January 2019 by authority of the House of Commons, UK.

The IFS Deaton Review (2020) Inequality [Online]. Available at: https://www.ifs.org.uk/inequality/about-the-review/ (Accessed: 14 July 2020).

Kessler et al. (2007) 'Lifetime prevalence and age-of-onset distributions of mental disorders in the World Health Organization's World Mental Health Survey Initiative', World Psychiatry, 2007(6), pp. 168–176.

Kramer, E. (1958) Art therapy in a children's community. Springfield: Charles C. Thomas.

Kramer, E. (1971) Art as therapy with children. New York: Schocken Books.

Kramer, E. (1979) Childhood and art therapy. New York: Schocken Books.

Kyu, H.H. et al. (May 2018) 'Causes of death among children aged 5–14 years in the WHO European Region: a systematic analysis for the Global Burden of Disease Study 2016', The Lancet, 2, 321-327. https://doi.org/10.1016/S2352-4642(18)30095-6.

Malhotra, S., and Sahoo, S. (2018) 'Antecedents of depression in children and adolescents', Industrial Psychiatry Journal, 27(1), 11–16.

Mandela, N. (1995) Speech by president Nelson Mandela at the launch of the Nelson Mandela Children's Fund, Mahlamba'ndlopfu, Pretoria, 8 May [Online]. Available at: https://www.sahistory.org.za/archive/speech-president-nelson-mandela-launch-nelson-mandela-childrens-fund-mahlambandlopfu (Accessed: 21 October 2020).

McDaniel, B.T., and Radesky, J. (2017) 'Technoference: Parent distraction by technology and associations with child behavior problems', Child Development [Online]. Available at: http://onlinelibrary.wiley.com/doi/10.1111/cdev.12822/full (Accessed: 29 June 2020).

National Scientific Council on the Developing Child (2015) Supportive relationships and active skill-building strengthen the foundations of resilience: Working Paper 13 [Online]. Available at: http://www.developingchild.harvard.edu (Accessed: 12 July 2020).

NHS (2018) Digital survey of the mental health of children and young people in England [Online]. Available at: https://digital.nhs.uk/data-and-information/publications/statistical/mental-health-of-children-and-young-people-in-england/2017/2017 (Accessed: 29 June 2020).

OECD (2018) *Children & young people's mental health in the digital age shaping the future* [Online]. Available at https://www.oecd.org/els/health-systems/Children-and-Young-People-Mental-Health-in-the-Digital-Age.pdf (Accessed: 29 June 2020).

OECD (2019) *Family database, social policy division, directorate of employment, labour and social affairs, CO2.2: Child poverty, November 2019* [Online]. Available at: http://www.oecd.org/els/family/database.htm (Accessed: 28 June 2020).

Ozer, S. (2019) 'Towards a psychology of cultural globalisation: A sense of self in a changing world', *Psychology & Developing Societies*, 31(1), pp. 162–186.

Raab, M., Ruland, M., Schonberger, B., Blossfeld, H.-P., Hofacker, D., Buchholz, S., and Schmelzer, P. (2008) 'GlobalIndex: A sociological approach to globalization measurement', *International Sociology*, 23, pp. 596–631.

Trent, M., Dooley, D.G., and Dougé, J. (2019) 'The impact of racism on child and adolescent health', *Pediatrics* 144 (2), pp. 1–14.

UNICEF (2017) *The adolescent brain: A second window of opportunity: A Compendium, Innocenti (2017)*. Florence: UNICEF Office of Research – Innocenti.

UNICEF (2019a) *For every child, every right, The Convention on the Rights of the Child at a crossroads* [Online]. Available at: https://www.unicef.org/reports/convention-rights-child-crossroads-2019 (Accessed: 3 July 2020).

UNICEF (2019b) *Increase in child and adolescent mental disorders spurs new push for action by UNICEF and WHO* [Online]. Available at: https://www.unicef.org/press-releases/increase-child-and-adolescent-mental-disorders-spurs-new-push-action-unicef-and-who (Accessed: 28 June 2020).

UNICEF 2020. *Measuring and monitoring child poverty, Position paper, March 2020* [Online]. Avaiable at: https://data.unicef.org/resources/measuring-and-monitoring-child-poverty/ (Accessed: 3 July 2020).

United Nations (2015) *Transforming our world: the 2030 Agenda for Sustainable Development* [Online]. Available at: https://www.un.org/ga/search/view_doc.asp?symbol=A/RES/70/1&Lang=E (Accessed: 1 November 2020).

WHO (2014a) *WHO calls for stronger focus on adolescent health*, 24 May [Online]. Available at: https://www.who.int/mediacentre/news/releases/2014/focus-adolescent-health/en/ (Accessed: 1 July 2020).

WHO (2014b) *Adolescence: neurodevelopmental changes* [Online]. Available at: https://apps.who.int/adolescent/second-decade/section2/page4/adolescence-neurodevelopmental-changes.html, (Accessed: 30 June 2020).

WHO (2017) *World Health Organization, Mental Health Atlas (2017)* [Online]. Available at: https://www.who.int/mental_health/evidence/atlas/mental_health_atlas_2017/en/ (Accessed: 26 June 2020).

WHO (2019a) *HEN-Health Evidence Network synthesis report 67, What is the evidence on the role of the arts in improving health and well-being? A scoping review (2019)* [Online]. Available at: https://www.euro.who.int/en/publications/abstracts/what-is-the-evidence-on-the-role-of-the-arts-in-improving-health-and-well-being-a-scoping-review-2019 (Accessed: 1 July 2020).

WHO (2019b) *Suicide, key facts* [Online]. Available at: https://www.who.int/news-room/fact-sheets/detail/suicide (Accessed: 30 June 2020).

WHO (2019c) *Adolescent mental health, key facts* [Online]. Available at: https://www.who.int/news-room/fact-sheets/detail/adolescent-mental-health (Accessed: 30 June 2020).

WHO, ICD 11 (2018) *Gaming disorder* [Online]. Available at: https://icd.who.int/browse11/l-m/en#/http://id.who.int/icd/entity/1448597234 (Accessed: 1 July 2020).

1

'BEANS OF HOPE' – BUILDING RESILIENCE THROUGH PLAY PSYCHOTHERAPY FOR YEAR-SIX PUPILS TRANSITIONING INTO SECONDARY SCHOOL

Di Gammage

> *'Resilience is the human capacity to face, overcome and be strengthened by or even transformed by adversities of life. Everyone faces adversities, no one is exempt ... With resilience, children can triumph over trauma; without it, trauma (adversity) triumphs.'*
>
> *(Grotberg, 1995, p.10)*
>
> *As a teacher you have to believe in your children – that anything is possible in their lives, however dire, desperate, barren they might be.*
>
> *– (Head teacher 'Beans of Hope' Primary School)*

Introduction

Psychotherapists know the impact of chronic stress on their clients anecdotally. This is supported by the negative impact of chronic stress on the cardio-physiology system (Porges, 1995), on the immune system (Benschop et al., 1994) and mental (Esch et al., 2002) and cognitive functioning. The CoC Programme, devised by Derek Roger (1995, 2002, 2005, 2007), is a proven effective intervention that benefits cardio-physiology (Roger, 1998). Although the programme is specific to adults in the workplace, and there is no reference to children in school, the author recognised a link between adult characteristics that support or compromise resilience to characteristics seen in children. Vulnerable children struggling with trauma, difficult relationships, and school pressures are more likely to engage in unhelpful ways of thinking that severely compromise their capacity to learn. Such habitual ways of thinking, defined as rumination (Roger, 1995), trigger a defensive reaction and, at times, the survival mechanism of fight-or-flight. As such times, it is extremely difficult to think clearly.

There are real dangers in life that demand a fight or flight reaction; however, hyperalert or hypervigilant children are much more likely to ruminate. Defensive ways of being are contagious and will have a negative impact on a child's learning, relationships with peers, and how they are viewed and experienced by teachers. The chapter's title, 'Beans of Hope', is based on an interaction between one of the children and the author that reflects children's capacity to adapt, learn and develop habits that support their emotional resilience, given the opportunities to do so. According to Becker (1997), resilience is considered the single most significant predictive factor in living a successful life beyond education, training and experience. With an increase in the number of primary-aged children in the UK being diagnosed with anxiety and depression (4% of children between the ages of 5 and 16) (Green et al., 2004) to around one in eight children aged 5 to 19 (Baker, 2020) and the established links of such mental health conditions to stress (Roger, 1995) resulting in ever-growing demands on child mental health services, attention must be given to prevention and early intervention.

For many children, primary education can provide a much-needed safe and predictable sanctuary. The transition to secondary education can be overwhelming and disorientating for the more vulnerable children. Furthermore, how children establish themselves in year, seven can set the trajectory for academic achievement and educational satisfaction.

This study's focus is a pilot study conducted by a therapist/researcher offered to year 6 pupils developed in conjunction with a new primary school. The school has three times the national average of children with an Education Health and Care Plan (EHCP) and a significantly higher ratio of children (information from school register) on the Child Protection Register than other primary schools in the county.

This was an action-based enquiry (Lewin, 1946; Robson, 2002), involving 16 children, in which the purpose of the intervention was to identify habitual factors that indicate children's levels of resilience before and after a 20-session programme in a small group setting drawing on a questionnaire based on the CoC Training Programme.

This chapter discusses the relationship between play and mindfulness and the role of these disciplines in building emotional resilience (Gammage, 2017). Play psychotherapy brings together the depth psychological understanding of child psychotherapy and well-established creative methods of play therapy, including story-making, role play, art and projective play. The four steps of the CoC programme were incorporated into the play psychotherapy through mindfulness exercises and relaxation. This chapter concludes with reflections on this pioneering study and draws recommendations for furthering emotional resilience work in primary schools.

Theoretical background

Resilience is understood to be linked to 'overcoming the odds, sustaining competence under pressure and recovery from trauma' (Fraser et al., 1999, p. 136). In the CoC programme, a clear distinction is made between *pressure* and *stress:* pressure is described as 'the demand to perform' and ranges from, for instance, getting out of bed in the morning when the alarm rings to sitting an exam; the CoC programme defines stress as rumination. In the CoC programme, emotional resilience is a skill which allows us to avoid turning pressure into stress. Individual characteristics, such as genetics contribute to emotional resilience (Werner, 1989); however, a significant factor is thesocial environment. There is still much debate around a definitive definition of resilience. It is recognised as a trait, process and outcome strongly influenced by a relationship as nature and nurture both play a part in the development of resilience. Crucially, resilience is not about blaming an individual or shifting the burden of responsibility onto the individual; in this context, the child, to change their life circumstances.

The Challenge of Change Resilience Programme©

The author, a play psychotherapist, is accredited to deliver the CoC programme. In the 1980s, whilst based in the Psychology Department at the University of York, academic Dr Derek Roger was invited to undertake research on resilience with North Yorkshire police amongst other organisations. Focusing on the question 'What is it that makes some people more vulnerable to stress and others more resilient?' he was able to recruit a number of doctoral students with the intention of identifying specific ways of thinking that either supported emotional resilience or, conversely, had a negative impact upon it. Roger and his students noted that these factors could be measured by monitoring the cardiovascular and immune systems, thus creating a body of knowledge based on empirical research that linked stress to the physical body and clearly showed the damaging effect of chronic stress on mental and physical health. Roger subsequently collated the individual studies devising a training programme which he called the CoC.

Mindfulness

The CoC programme is fundamentally a mindfulness programme. According to Flood 2017, sales of books relating to mindfulness rose by 13% in that year against a backdrop of falling book sales in practically every other genre. A well-known online bookseller is currently offering over a hundred titles of mindfulness books and activities for children and adolescents. It seems we are desperately eager to pursue mindfulness for ourselves and our offspring and perhaps for a good reason. Lama Surya Das observes, 'Learning to maintain mindfulness and perspective when we are facing personal upheaval is extraordinarily relevant to modern times' (1997, p. 372). Yet Roger would ask us to consider the question, 'What is your mind full of?' What is key is being able to recognise certain habitual ways of thinking and to be able to take charge of our minds. The CoC programme is simple, but it is not easy because old ways of thinking are ingrained and tenacious. Being able to control our minds is a moment-to-moment practicThe aspect of taking charge of our own minds, and in particular the area of self-regulation, was a core feature of the Beans of Hope project. Self-regulation is understood as the ability to respond to a situation with socially acceptable emotional reactions and to be able to inhibit emotions that lead to unacceptable behaviours. In order to self-regulate emotionally, it is necessary both to recognise and to calm one's emotions. One of the most comprehensive longitudinal psychological studies carried out strongly suggests that early childhood emotional self-control is a significant predictor in mental, physical and social wellbeing in adults (Moffitt et al., 2011).

The inevitability of change

The programme is called the CoC because, mostly, as long as life is stable, predictable, and safe, we generally manage well. The challenge is when we experience change, especially change we ourselves do not initiate and/or feel we have little choice in influencing. Change is an inevitable aspect of life. It can be both exciting and fear-provoking, presenting new opportunities and new challenges (Coffey, 2009, 2013). The shift from primary to secondary school can be a shocking, lonely and isolating experience, due to the differences in culture and size of the school and expectations placed upon children (Ganeson, 2006). Children are required to adapt and cope as they face these significant changes as well as losing the relative intimacy of their primary school and established relationships with teachers, auxiliary staff and sometimes friendships. Primary and secondary schools have increasingly collaborated to support children in making this 'rite of passage' (Pratt and George, 2005), so called transition programmes. (Ganeson, 2006) inline with a growing body of evidence, suggesting that early disengagement can lead to poorer academic success, school attendance and increased antisocial behaviour (Chadbourne, 2001; Daly et al., 2009; Rudzinskas, 2008). Levels of stress are observed even in children who successfully navigate this transition (Roeser and Eccles, 1998).

The four steps of the Challenge of Change Resilience Programme©

There are four steps in the CoC Resilience Programme – Waking up and Staying Awake, Focusing Attention, Detaching and Letting go. 'Waking sleep' is a term coined by Roger to describe a state of being awake still, not in the present moment, an example of which would be driving the car but having one's mind on the meeting just attended, or about to be attended, or sitting in a classroom and staring out of the window watching the clouds go by. Being in a state of waking sleep is not stressful per se; however, if one is not present behind the wheel of a car, one could argue that there are significant potential risks involved that could easily result in dire consequences. Waking sleep is the place of daydreaming which can at times be a highly enjoyable and productive pastime. It entirely depends on the circumstances. In the classroom example, the child will miss the teacher's instruction, not know what to do and possibly be identified as time-wasting or badly behaved. Besides the obvious risks involved in ill-timed waking sleep, when we are in this state of mind, we are clearly not in the present moment and thus are unable to control where we place our attention. In waking sleep, our attention can be snatched away by any whim. These might be quite harmless and of little or no consequence, or the daydream can become a nightmare as we begin to ruminate on past events or future imagined events. In the nightmare, these are accompanied by powerful upsetting feelings. This is rumination and one of the core factors understood to adversely affect our emotional resilience. These are the *if onlys* and *what ifs* that occupy many minds that can lead to depression and anxiety, respectively.

It is only when we are truly awake that we are able to control where we place our attention. From this state of being wide awake, we can stop ourselves disappearing down the rabbit hole of past events that cannot be changed. Many people confuse rumination with reflection: they believe themselves to be problem-solving when in effect they are dwelling on unresolved issues in habitual patterns of thought or worrying about events that may or may not take place in the future. It is extremely difficult to think clearly when we are being bombarded with angry or upsetting emotions.

Detachment, that quality of putting things into perspective, is the third step of the CoC programme and understood to be one of the most valuable factors in developing emotional resilience and therefore, included in the psychometric assessment known as the Profile.

The fourth step of the CoC programme is Letting go. This means letting go of the ruminative thoughts and accompanying emotions that prevent us from having that presence of mind and being able to employ the WIN technique (What's Important Now) as we are only able to give our attention to one task at a time (excluding the tiny minority of individuals known to possess a super brain).

Play

Play brings us into the present moment. We can only play in the 'here-and-now', and presence of mind is an essential aspect of play. As true play has a focus on the process rather than the product or end result, it is a natural antidote to 'Toxic Achieving' – one of the factors recognised in the CoC to seriously compromise emotional resilience. According to Panksepp (2004), opioids and dopamine are activated during playful interactions. These powerful chemicals suppress pain and distress and promote feelings of enjoyment and pleasure. Play is also known to stimulate the higher, 'upstairs' regions of the brain responsible for cognitive and reflective functioning (Panksepp, 2004; Pellis and Pellis, 2006). An important aspect of resilience is recognising what is and is not within our power to change, according to Kernberg (in Knowlton, 2001), play is a powerful medium for healing as a child can control, formulate and change the events of his or her play. In play psychotherapy, it is possible to process or metabolise a traumatic event and transform one's relationship to that event in the present.

The play opportunities made available to the children in the Beans of Hope Project included embodiment, projective and role play. The three stages are known as the Developmental Play Paradigm (Jennings, 1999). Embodiment play relating directly to body and senses was supported by activities such as mindful breathing, clay work and work through gesture. Projective play was addressed through exercises that included identifying metaphors to describe emotional states, drawing, story-making and storytelling, and role play was used by the children to enact the stories they had written.

Design

This was an action-based enquiry (Lewin, 1946; Robson, 2002). However, there was also a spiral quality to it – that is, discovery, planning, reflection and then more discovery, planning and reflection with the research feeding back directly to the process. Thus, there were also aspects of a group case study enquiry (Kraft, 2012). Action-based research is a method intended to improve practice –, adult inter-actions with children – enabling the children to feel more empowered, more confident, and better equipped to make decisions that will support their in-tegration into secondary school. The model involves action, evaluation and critical reflection resulting in changes in practice being implemented. An action-based approach suited this research. It offered a participatory and collaborative model, which encouraged the children to reflect on the work, share these reflections with the facilitators, and witness integration of their ideas and thoughts. It was essential that the facilitators worked from the basis of hearing and respecting the children's voices, and that the contributions of the children were acknowledged (Jones and Welch, 2018).

The purpose of the intervention was to support the child-participants' devel-opment of key factors identified by the Coc Programme. The intervention took place in three groups of four pupils per group over a period of 20 weeks. Each session lasted for 50 minutes. The author facilitated the groups supported by an assistant in 10 of the 20 sessions over alternate weeks with the 10 intervening sessions being led by one of two assistants. The purpose behind alternating the sessions was to allow the children to practice the new habits they were being introduced to, consolidate their learning, reflect, and offer feedback. In two of the groups, the assistant was a school teaching assistant and a trainee play therapist in the remaining group.

The groups were selected in conjunction with the head teacher and the two year-six classroom teachers who knew the children and their needs. It was decided that each group would comprise two boys and two girls. Twelve further children were randomly chosen as the control group. These children did not take part in the sessions.

A questionnaire was used before and following the intervention that focused on the eight key factors identified as supporting or impeding emotional resilience. These factors are understood to be largely habitual and learned behaviour and thus, with awareness and practice, can be developed or minimised. The questionnaire was compiled using the existing body of empirical research that underpins the

CoC resilience programmeincludes measures of resilience using a rating scale. All children taking part in the intervention and the children in the control group were asked to complete the questionnaire before and after the intervention and the lead researcher/facilitator collated the results.

Parents were invited to attend a parental session led by the author and the head teacher. This meeting's purpose was to explain key aspects of the intervention so that parents could understand and support any new language the children may adopt.

Each child in the Project was interviewed for 20 minutes individually around 15 weeks into the project. The children were encouraged to reflect on the work so far, invited to give feedback and any suggestions or thoughts for the remaining sessions. These interviews were documented and shared between the three facilitators, and the children's ideas informed the running of the ongoing groups.

The questionnaire

The Beans of Hope Project comprised a 14-point questionnaire created using the expert opinions of the head teacher and class teachers to ensure using child-friendly language evoking information relating to self-image, confidence in one's ability to problem-solve, trust in adults for comfort and help, peer relationships, tolerance of mistakes, flexibility (to manage change) and willingness to meet challenges. Children were asked to grade themselves from 1 to 10 where 1 was Not at All and 10 was Always. The children were also invited to use three words to describe themselves, three words they thought their parents/carers would use, three words their teacher would use and three words their friends would use to describe them.

The first question asked of the children, 'How much do you like yourself?' relates to self-esteem which develops from experiences and situations that have influenced how one sees oneself. The question 'How happy are you with your life?' seeks to elicit the children's degree of contentment with their lives.

In the Beans of Hope questionnaire, specific questions relating to dependency on adults were asked, for example, 'How much can you trust that adults will be able to support and help you in your life?', 'How confident are you that you can turn to someone when you are upset?' and 'If you are worried how likely are you to ask for help?'. Issues of trust, confidence in others and seeking out others for comfort are relevant in adults' lives; however, there is recognition given to children's greater dependency on adults (parents, teachers, carers and possibly siblings) to support them. Detached Coping is addressed in the questions, 'How often do good things happen in your life?', and 'Do you think it is inevitable that bad things will happen in life?' and Perfect Control with the question, 'Is it OK to make mistakes?'.

Emotional resilience is understood as the ability to cope with adversity and to be able to adapt to change. Coping with adversity and recognising one's personal sense of agency (self-confidence) are addressed in many of the questions but most specifically by, 'How confident are you about your own abilities to deal with life?', 'How much do you believe problems and difficulties can be solved?', 'How much do you enjoy challenging yourself?' and 'How well do you cope when things don't go according to plan?'. The quality of Flexibility is also addressed by the last of these questions.

Finally, the children were asked, 'How much do you care what other people think of you?'. This question sought to reveal the children's dependence on other people and was inspired by Carl Rogers' concept of the locus of evaluation (2003). The locus of evaluation relates to a person's dependence or independence on others' judgment for appraisal and approval of themselves. Where the locus is external in adults, there is deemed to be an overreliance on others' opinions, guidance and advice; however, in the case of 10 and 11 year olds, one would anticipate their being a degree of externalisation particularly in relation to parents/carers and teachers.

Prior to the CoC one-day training, participants are asked to complete an online psychometric assessment, the Profile, based on the accrued research mentioned earlier.

Unlike the Profile, the Beans of Hope questionnaire was not compiled directly from research. Rather, it was informed by the eight factors identified in the CoC assessment. As stated earlier, the Profile relates specifically to adults within a workplace setting so the factors outlined earlier needed to be considered in relation to children within a school setting. In the Profile, there are five factors understood to undermine our capacity to be emotionally resilient – Rumination (a preoccupation with past events or imagined future events accompanied by an upsetting emotion such as anger, fear, worry or distress), Perfect Control (an inability to recognise when something is 'good enough', also defined as perfectionism), Emotional Inhibition (repression of upsetting emotions), Toxic Achieving (an over-focus on the end result with a disregard for how that is achieved) and Avoidance Coping. There are three factors recognised as contributing to emotional resilience – Detached Coping (putting things into perspective/not making a mountain out of a mole hill), Sensitivity (attunement to other people's emotional states) and Flexibility (ability to cope with chance). The questions compiled for the school questionnaire at times address more than one resilience factor.

The sessions

The facilitators sought to create a safe, non-threatening space for the children with time for them to listen to each other and to speak about their own life experiences. To talk about their worries and fears without that provoking any action from an adult was a key feature of these groups and noted by a number of the children in individual interviews. They did not wish for their material to be shared and acted upon (the issue of confidentiality in relation to child protection was discussed in initial sessions), rather, they needed a space in which to talk, explore, reflect and process. Several children also noted that by having this space without risk of adults sharing outside, one boy described as, 'other people trying to sort out my problems', communicated to the children that they had the capacity to problem-solve for themselves. As a consequence of this the children felt more empowered.

Each of the groups created their own agreement that included the values they held, their wishes and desires for the twenty sessions. They also designed their own group shield, together with a motto and a personalised name, that reflected their own personalities. In constructing their quarter of the group's shield, each child used drawing and words to represent aspects of themselves. This felt to be a very important aspect in establishing the overall ethos and practice for the Beans of Hope project to convey to the children that these were their groups and could influence what happens in the groups. For children of 10 and 11, especially in a school setting, this was a completely different experience, even in a school as child-oriented as the host school.

The project children did not need to achieve any external goals, rather they were invited repeatedly to explore their own personal goals. However, it was necessary to offer the groups a structure that could provide holding and containment for them. This came in the form of opening with a standing circle, saying hello however they wished (verbally and/or physically) and focusing on breathing. This allowed all to be present within their bodies and let the group know how everyone was feeling. In order to support the children (and adults) in naming emotional states, the teaching assistant, who was also trained as an Emotional Literacy Support Assistant, provided a chart of emoji faces each showing a different emotion. Each group member could use the chart to identify their own feelings. As the sessions progressed, the assistant introduced a more comprehensive list of emotional states (without the emojis) and made those available to the groups. This list became especially useful when the House of the Mind was introduced to the children and they were seeking to populate the Upstairs and Downstairs Minds (explained further). The facilitators also introduced metaphors to help describe and share emotional states, such as, 'If we were a weather condition what would we be?' A white mist, scorching sunshine without any shade and a turbulent storm at sea with no safe harbour, were shared ideas. Including metaphors such as these allowed group members to understand that play does not necessarily have to be embodied and physicalised. It can be images shared verbally that can be recreated in others' minds. In a subsequent session, the trainee play therapist introduced the metaphor of a fizzy pop bottle and twisting the top a little at a time to illustrate the practices of titration and pendulation. Titration is the processing of slowing down one's response to an event, in particular a traumatic event, so that one can control how much is manageable at that time. Pendulation is the act of moving towards an experience of activation caused by trauma and away from it back into a place of resource. Once resourced, one can then move back slowly and in control (using titration) to the traumatic material. These are deeply empowering exercises as they much reduce the risk of overwhelm and retraumatisation. Both of these therapeutic processes are taken from Somatic Experiencing therapy also known as the Trauma Resiliency Model developed by Peter Levine (Levine, 2010).

As the groups warmed up over the ensuing weeks and began to talk excitedly about their experiences and thoughts, we collectively decided to introduce the equivalent of a talking stick in the shape of a wooden heart. The children thoroughly enjoyed this practice and showed impressive levels of self-governance. They would frequently make a big show of silence (fingers across sealed lips), enthusiastically pointing to the wooden heart. Others would helpfully pass it to the speaker-to-be. There were no incidents of children withholding or being possessive of the wooden heart.

One of the project's main focuses was to help the children understand better what is happening in their brains so that they might feel more empowered to practice control and make choices. To this end, we introduced an exercise called 'The Brain House: Upstairs and Downstairs' derived from the work of Siegel and Payne Bryson (2012) by Hazel Harrison (2018). Harrison has created a dramatic, interactive and playful model based on the functions of the neocortex (the thinking brain: the upstairs) and the limbic system (the feeling brain: the downstairs) by asking children to consider which characters live upstairs and which characters downstairs. The downstairs characters' purpose is fundamentally to keep one safe by ensuring needs are met. These characters are alert to danger – physical and psychological – and where there has been trauma, they may well be in a state of hypervigilance. In such an event, without the more considered, rational, thoughtful and detached characters from upstairs, the downstairs folk will quickly become dysregulated and likely then that the Big Red Button (i.e. the amygdala) will be pressed.

Children draw their own brain house and add a variety of characters, for instance, Calming Caroline, Problem-Solving Pete and Flexible Fred living upstairs whilst the downstairs is inhabited by Frightened Frieda, Worried William and Angry Andy. The two floors are connected by a flight of stairs so that upstairs characters are able to comfort and regulate the dysregulated downstairs characters. Also living downstairs is one particular character who Harrison refers to as Big Boss Bootsy. Big Boss' job is to press the Big Red Button if situations become dangerous. When the Button is pressed, the Lid is Flipped (a phrase used by Dan Siegel), the floors become disconnected and the downstairs characters take over. Once the children had drawn their own versions of inhabitants in the groups, discussions ensued as to when Flipping the Lid would be the safest course of action.

Neurologically, adolescence extends until approximately 24 years and so these children's brains are far from maturity (Siegel, 2013); however, by the age of 10 and 11, the children's neocortex brains are noticeably present. They were able to listen to each other, reflect, empathise and make suggestions to one another on numerous occasions. When a child is Flipping their Lid, then it is for the adults around to 'lend' them their intact brains (to regulate on the child's behalf) until the child's Upstairs and Downstairs brains are reconnected. For some children, of course, they will have direct experience of the adults in their lives flipping their own lids and sometimes the children themselves have needed to take on the role of regulator to adults.

The children then wrote their own short scripts that depicted situations in which Big Bossy Bootsy pressed the Big Red Button prematurely (causing mayhem). Together, they created role plays, taking on these characters, stopping the action and consulting with the Upstairs characters. The facilitators supported the children's exploration, asking questions, taking on roles if required, but generally taking a backstage role so that the children could lead their own dramas. Sometimes, Big Boss Bootsy did resort to the Button, but other times the children seemed able to navigate their own journeys with each other's help and suggestions.

Sometimes, one child would lend one of their own characters to another child's Upstairs Brain. The degree of self-regulation in executing the exercise itself was impressive and reflected upon by the children afterwards. They seemed to have surprised themselves by their own capacity.

Another House exercise was introduced to the groups, borrowed from the CoC programme. This is the House of the Mind in which all thoughts can be seen flooding into the house as if through a flapping door. We have no way of controlling these thoughts and they can be overwhelming. This state corresponds to waking sleep(mentioned earlier).

The children were set a task. How could we stay in the House of our Minds, still allowing those thoughts to come in (since ultimately, we cannot stop them) but not become overwhelmed and end up drowning in them? Some children worked out that it would be necessary to 'get to higher ground'. They created an attic/loft space they could retreat to and, crucially, opened up the ground floor space to allow the thoughts and memories with accompanying feelings to flow through. From their vantage point, they can see those passing through without being caught up in them. This is the place of 'super-vision', detached coping and being wide awake. There is also a strong resonance between the House of the Mind model and the Upstairs and Downstairs Brain.

In one session, the children were invited to work with clay in silence. The facilitators were initially unsure how the children would respond to this, especially working individually and without words. Remarkably, many of the children chose to close their eyes often for several minutes at a time so that they could experience the texture of the clay without focusing on what they were making with it. This was pure embodiment play for these children and several of them commented that they would like an additional clay session. This was organised due to popular demand.One child created a coffin after attending a relative's funeral during the life of the project. She chose to share her sculpture with her group and talk about her feelings of sadness at his loss and its impact on her mother. Other children chose to beat, flatten, fold and roll their clay without any fixed outcome.

In the ending sessions, the groups and facilitators celebrated with cupcakes and balloons. The children delighted in blowing up the balloons and letting them go, giggling at their erratic behaviour and rude noises. They tied them and created their own games, including play fighting and more sport-orientated exercises. The facilitators took part, at the children's invitation.

Besides everything else, it was hoped that these sessions would allow the children to have fun, laugh together, share, work, and play together. It felt like the final balloon and cake session epitomised this aim.

Results

Prior to the project's commencement, the 12 children selected to take part plus 12 children identified as the control group were invited to fill in the questionnaire. A member of staff was present to clarify any questions the children did not understand. Following the 20 sessions, the same children, in the same format, reset the questionnaires. All information was collated, scored and analysed. Follow-up questionnaire scores were added up from 0 to 10 relating to each question and compared to initial questionnaire scores. The control and intervention groups' scores were then compared to each other.

All 12 children consistently attended all 20 sessions except one boy who missed one due to ill-health. Throughout the project, all the children appeared interested to take part and this eagerness grew as they became more visibly relaxed over the course of the project.

Eight mothers attended the first parental session and responded with interest and enthusiasm to the project. It was apparent during this meeting that the women were supportive and empathic towards one another, suggesting a support network beyond the school setting.

In the first questionnaire, the control group children scored marginally higher than project groups on self-esteem, trust that adults would be able to support and help, and friendship groups. The control group children scored significantly higher on confidence in their own abilities to deal with life in the first questionnaire than the project group children. On all other questions, there were no measurable differences between the groups.

On the follow-up questionnaire, the project groups showed noticeable change compared to their pre-project questionnaire in the area of confidence in their own abilities to deal with life. Their follow-up results rated higher than the control group results which had not changed from the first questionnaire. Coupled with this, the project group children scored a significant increase in their belief that good things often happen in their lives. This increase was smaller than the increase in the belief that bad things were inevitable in life. Good and bad things arising are not necessarily the problem, it is one's capacity to deal with them. In the control group, there was no noticeable change in either of these scores.

The project group children's score overall in response to the question about making mistakes was particularly apparent with seven children increasing their score, three remaining the same and two children scoring themselves lower on the follow-up questionnaire. The higher score denotes an acceptance of the inevitability of making mistakes. By contrast, in the control group children, eight children's scores remained unchanged, three had increased and one fallen. Overall, the control group children scored higher on the pre-project questionnaires but in the follow-up questionnaires, the project group children rated the same and slightly higher than the control group children on the question of making mistakes.

There was no change in the control group children's scores between their first and second questionnaire results on the question of challenging themselves. In the project group, seven children rated more enjoyment in challenging themselves, one remained the same and three had marginally reduced scores; however, overall the project group children rated higher than the control group children on the follow-up questionnaire.

In response to the question relating to caring what others thought about them, a lower score might denote greater independence/self-esteem/less reliance on the opinions of others' for self-validation. In the project group children, there was a significant increase between initial and follow-up questionnaires in relation to the question of caring what other people thought of them. This was in marked contrast to the control group children who initially scored marginally higher than the project group children and whose scores changed only minimally in the follow-up questionnaires.

There were very noticeable differences between the control and project groups in the language used to describe themselves and how they believe others would describe them. There were no differences between the number of times children described themselves and believed others would describe them, as 'funny', 'kind', 'naughty', 'friendly', 'chatty' and 'crazy'. However, the control group children selected words such as 'supportive', 'kind-hearted', 'confident', empathetic', 'good-mannered', 'a bit hot-headed', 'enthusiastic', 'committed', 'unique', 'adventurous' and 'sophisticated' and language that may be viewed as more complex. Although the project group children often referred to themselves as 'smart', 'cool', 'silly' and 'thoughtful', their descriptions related far more frequently to their physical appearance such as, 'ugly', 'tall' and 'good hair'. They also more frequently described their unhappiness and upsetting emotions such as 'anger' and 'feeling alone'.

In the mid-project interviews, the children shared the following reflections:

> 'I've loved having a voice – if you don't have a voice you feel powerless'.
> 'I've seen changes in my own and my friends' behaviour – for the better!'
> 'Hearing how it is for other people…it's made me grateful for my own mum and dad'.
> 'Resilience is coping with things you can't change – and being gentle with yourself'.
> 'When I first came to this school, I used to get angry because I missed my old friends. I've made new ones now (I still miss my old ones, but I don't get angry so much anymore)'
> 'I have a saying – am I living to die, or dying to live?'
> 'I realised just how much I used to overthink'.
> 'I LOVED the clay session – with my eyes closed and being in silence'.
> 'I like the WIN (What's Important Now?)'.
> 'We all got better at being friends in the group'.
> 'I like the rule – what's said in the room, stays in the room. It makes me feel safe'.
> 'I was surprised because often adults make it worse!'

Analysis and reflections

As the project children were specifically selected in view of their particular difficulties identified in the classroom and their increased vulnerability, it follows that these children showed consistently lower scores on self-esteem, self-confidence, trust in adults' support and poor peer relationships. Prior to the project, these children registered as generally less empowered that the children selected to be part of the control group.

The Beans of Hope children were identified by their teachers as more vulnerable than their peers, struggling with relationships and with emotional regulation. It is possible that these children would also be assessed as having insecure attachment patterns with their primary carers. Many of these children will have experienced neglect and abuse in their lives, even if those were not current at the time of the project. It is likely that these children will have learned from an early age that emotions, particularly powerful emotions, are frightening as they will have witnessed them in the adults around them. In addition, the children may not have had a safe other to give them comfort at times of their own distress. A child's ability to explore their world safely is significantly hindered in the absence of a safe system in the home environment. For such children, their ability to regulate their emotions is reduced and distrust affects their ability to make connections with others (Blaustein and Kinniburgh, 2019).

There was a significant increase in the Beans of Hope children's scores between the initial questionnaire and follow-up in relation to the question of caring what other people thought of them. Initially, the author regarded this result as a negative one illustrating these children's further reliance on others for approval. A different perspective arose in discussion with her supervisor on other possible reasons for the marked increase in these scores. It could reflect an increase in sensitivity if the children had paid more attention to the wording, 'caring what other people thought'. It may also be helpful to explore in the sessions themselves how the children understood the meaning of the word 'care'. A child's response to this question could demonstrate a more relational way of being for these children. Trosclair (2015) recognises our nature as social animals and 'needing to be liked enough as part of the tribe has been highly adaptive for our survival as a species' (2015, p. 12). Providing the children did not become overreliant on the approval of others and were able to develop a healthy interdependence on others would surely support them as they progress to secondary school and forge new relationships with peers and teachers. This may also signify a positive step for these children to build more trusting relationships with adults and children. This was evidenced in the statement, 'We all got better at being friends in the group'.

Most of the project children were understood by the teachers to be hypervigilant and employ defensive ways of behaving and thinking. The phrase, 'it wasn't me', was very common when behavioural difficulties arose in the classroom or playground. Difficulty in taking responsibility for self and one's actions for some children is far too threatening as it can easily trigger shame. Shame is certainly something to defend against because it is distressing, painful and humiliating and quite likely to lead to punishment and expulsion from group. It was essential that these children experience an environment of non-judgement created by the adults that would allow for curiosity, self-acceptance and exploration without fear of being wrong. The safe environment was evidenced by such statements as, 'I like the rule – what's said in the room, stays in the room. It makes me feel safe' and, 'I was surprised because often adults make it worse!' There was a significant increase in the first and second questionnaire rating in the project children's belief in self-confidence relating to their own abilities to deal with life. As noted earlier, there was no change in the control children's rating on this question. This would suggest that the project children experienced a level of acceptance within the group modelled by the facilitators that allowed them to take charge of their own behaviour, thoughts and ideas and try them out without fear of rejection or failure. Certainly, the children's enthusiasm in all activities strongly indicated this.

One of the project's main focuses was to help the children better understand what was happening in their brains so that they might feel more empowered to practice control and make choices. One boy's reflective comment, 'I realised just how much I used to overthink' illustrates an ability to view himself in a detached way, evaluate this, and actively begin to curb this overthinking (rumination). The same boy arrived at a rather profound state of mind, exclaiming, 'I question myself – am I living to die, or dying to live?'

This was a very short-term study spanning only 20 sessions. We will not know the project's long-term impact as the study is not longitudinal and there was no follow-up with the children once they had transitioned into secondary school. As this was an action-based enquiry with a spiral quality comprising discovery, planning, reflection followed by further discovery, planning and reflection, it would be worthwhile to meet with the same twelve children in year seven, their first year of secondary school, to reflect more on the Beans of Hope Project. In order to develop this research further, it would be advantageous to create a questionnaire, similar to the CoC profile, using direct speech from participants and undertake a depth analysis of the findings. Unfortunately, this was not possible with this project; however, it is hoped that the outcome from this modest project will provide inspiration for other emotional resilience work with children.

At the beginning of this chapter, the author posed the question of whether it was ethical to seek to cultivate children's emotional resilience in such a project as the Beans of Hope. The author would conclude that doing nothing to support such children is itself unethical.

Reflecting on the children's verbal and written feedback throughout and at the end of the Beans of Hope Project, it was apparent that they enjoyed the time spent together. They had had novel experiences together and felt privileged to have taken part. This chapter began with a quote from their head teacher, an individual who truly believed and held hope for the children in her care and practised what she preached in the school. She was a leader from 'the back', supporting and encouraging her teaching and auxiliary staff to believe in the children. It was her idea to initiate this project and seek the funding to make it happen. It is to her, the assistants and classroom teachers and especially to the children who so willingly and fully engaged in this project, that this chapter is dedicated.

References

Baker, C. (2020) 'Mental health statistics for England: prevalence, services and funding', *House of Commons Library*, 6988, 23 January.

Becker, D. (1997) 'Adaptive Learning' Available at: http://www.adaptivlearningcom (Accessed 21 January 2021).

Benschop, R.J., Brosschot, J.F., Godaert, M.B., De Smet, M.D., Geenen, R., Olff, M., Heijnen, C.J., and Ballieux, R.E. (1994) 'Chronic stress affects immunologic but not cardiovascular responsiveness to acute psychological stress in humans' *American Journal of Physiology-Regulatory, Integrative and Comparative* Physiology, 226(1), pp. R75–R80.

Blaustein, M., and Kinniburgh, K.M. (2019) *Treating traumatic stress in children and adolescents: How to foster resilience through attachment, self-regulation and competency.* 2nd edn. New York: Guilford Press.

Chadbourne, R. (2001) *Middle schooling for the middle years: What might the jury be considering?* Southbank, VIC: Australian Education Union.

Coffey, A. (2009) 'Managing the move', ResearchOnline@ND. University of Notre Dame, Australia. Available at: https://researchonline.nd.edu.au/edu_article/48/ (Accessed: 7 January 2021).

Coffey, A. (2013) 'Relationships: The key to successful transition from primary to secondary school?', *Improving Schools,* 16(3), pp. 261–271.

Daly, B.P., Shin, R.Q., Thakral, C., Selders, M. and Vera, E. (2009) 'School engagement among urban adolescents of color: Does perception of social support and neighbourhood safety really matter?', *Journal of Youth Adolescence,* 38, pp. 63–74.

Das, S. (1997) *Awakening the buddha within.* New York: Broadway Books.

Esch, T., Stefano, G.B., Fricchione, G.L., and Benson, H. (2002) 'The role of stress in neurodegenerative diseases and mental disorders', *Neuroendocrinology Letters,* 23(3), pp. 199–208.

Flood, A. (2017) 'Sales of mind, body, spirit books boom in UK amid "mindfulness mega-trend"', *The Guardian,* 31 July.

Fraser, M., Richman, J., and Galinsky, M. (1999) 'Risk, protection and resilience: Toward a conceptual framework for social work practice', *Social Work* Research, 23(3), pp. 131–143.

Gammage, D. (2017) *Playful awakening – Releasing the gift of play in your life.* London: Jessica Kingsley Publications.

Ganeson, K. (2006). *Students' lived experience of transition into high school: A phenomenological study.* Unpublished doctoral dissertation, Queensland University of Technology, Brisbane, Australia. Eprints.qut.edu.au accessed 2/1/2020

Green, H. et al. (2004) *Mental health of children & young people in Great Britain.* Basingstoke: Palgrave Macmillan.

Grotberg, E. (1995) *A guide to promoting resilience in children: Strengthening the human spirit.* The International Resilience Project and the Bernard Van Leer Foundation, The Netherlands.

Harrison, H. (2018) How to Teach Kids about the Brain, Available at: www.mindful-org/how-to-teach-your-kids-about-the-brain (Accessed: 4 January 2020)

Jennings, S. (1999) *Introduction to developmental playtherapy.* London: Jessica Kingsley Publishers.

Jones, P., and Welch, S. (2018), *Rethinking children's rights – Attitudes in contemporary society.* 2nd edn. London: Bloomsbury.

Knowlton, L. (2001) 'The resilience of children in the face of trauma', *Psychiatric Times,* 17, 48–51.

Kraft, R.G. (2012) 'Group-inquiry turns passive students active' *Journal of College Science Teaching,* 33 (1985 – Issue 4, Published online 28 Aug 2012), 149–154.

Levine, P.A. (2010) *In an unspoken voice.* Berkeley, California: North Atlantic Books.

Lewin, K. (1946) Action research and minority problems. *Journal of Social Issues,* 2, pp. 34–36.

Mizelle, N.B. (2005) 'Moving out of middle school', *Educational Leadership,* 62(7), pp. 56–60.

Moffitt, T., Arseneault, L., Belsky, D., Dickson, N., Hancox, R.J., Harrington, H., Houts, R., Poulton, R., Roberts, B.W., Ross, S., Sears, M.R., Thompson, W.M., and Caspi, A. (2011) 'A gradient of childhood self-control predicts health, wealth, and public safety', *Proceedings of the National Academy of Sciences of the United States of* America, 108(7), pp. 2693–2698.

Olsson, C.A., Bond, L., Burns, J.M., Vella-Brodrick, D.A., and Sawyer, S.M. (2003) 'Adolescent resilience: A concept analysis', *Journal of Adolescence,* 26, pp. 1–11.

Panksepp, J. (2004) 'Emerging neuroscience of fear and anxiety: Therapeutic practice and clinical implications' in Panksepp, J. (ed.) *Textbook of biological psychiatry.* Hoboken, New Jersey: Wiley-Liss, pp. 489–512.

Pellis, S.M., and Pellis, V.C. (2006) 'Play and the development of social engagement: A comparative perspective' in Marshall, P. and Fox, N. (eds.) *The development of social engagement.* New York: OUP, pp. 247–274.

Porges, S. (1995) 'Cardiac vagal tone: A physiological index of stress', *Neuroscience & Biobehavioral* Reviews, 19(2), pp. 225–233.

Pratt, S., and George, R. (2005) 'Transferring friendship: Girls' and boys' friendships in the transition from primary to secondary school', *Children & Society,* 19, pp. 16–26.

Public Health England (December 2016). *The mental health of children and young people in England.* London: Wellington House.

Robson, C. (1993, 2002) *Real world research.* 2nd edn. Oxford: Blackwell Publishing.

Roeser, R.W., and Eccles, J.S. (1998) 'Adolescents' perceptions of middle school: Relation to longitudinal changes in academic and psychological adjustment', *Journal of Research on Adolescence,* 8(1), pp. 123–158.

Roger, D. (1995, 2002, 2005, 2007) *The challenge of change resilience programme.* New Zealand: The Work Skills Centre.

Roger, D. (April, 1998). 'The relationship between emotional rumination and cortisol under stress', *Individiual Differences,* 24(4), pp. 531–538.

Rogers, C. (2003). *Client-centred therapy.* London: Constable & Robinson.

Rudzinskas, A. (2008) 'Are middle years students unique?', *Australian Journal of Middle Schooling,* 8(2), pp. 24–26.

Schoon, I. (2006) *Risk and resilience: Adaptations in changing times.* Cambridge: Cambridge University Press.

Siegel, D. (2013) *Brainstorm: The power and purpose of the teenage brain.* New York: Jeremy P. Tarcher/Penguin.

Siegel, D., and Payne Bryson, T. (2012) *The whole-brain child.* New York: Bantam, Penguin Random House.

Trosclair, G. (2015) *I'm working on it in therapy.* New York: Skyhorse Publishing.

Werner, E.E. (1989) High-risk children in young adulthood: A longitudinal study from birth to 32 years. *American Journal of Orthopsychiatry,* 59(1), pp. 72–81. Available at: https:// www.hg.org/legal-articles/fatal-car-accident-statistics-29836 (Accessed: 4 January 2020) PMID: 2467566

2

BRIDGING PARENTS WITH THEIR CHILDREN WITH AUTISM IN MUSIC THERAPY – THE MUSIC-ORIENTED PARENT COUNSELLING MODEL

Tali Gottfried

In my clinical and research work, I often reflect on the unique contribution that music therapy has to offer to families of children with autism. While shared enjoyment and pleasure are natural ingredients in the parent–child relationship, pinned at the early stages of life and evolving throughout the years, they might be more complicated between parents and their children with autism. The unique characteristics of autism play a significant role in shaping the relationships formed within families of children with autism. Music therapy offers a way to interact in a simple and joyful way, planting the seeds to synchronicity and closeness. In order to establish a secure therapeutic alliance, the music therapist needs to be able to relate to the child and the parents in terms of frames, times and attunement. This chapter presents an evidence-based clinical model in music therapy, combining separate but parallel treatment of the child and the parents, which is called Music-Oriented Parent Counselling (MOPC). Theoretical perspectives will be reviewed alongside with therapeutic approaches, and a clinical vignette will illustrate one way to implement this model.

The setting – Parallel/Simultaneous treatment approach

Guided by the will to share and cooperate with parents through and with music, the Music-Oriented Parent Counselling (MOPC) model focuses on using music for the benefit of the child and the whole family. This model is rooted within my extensive clinical and research experience, and builds upon the *Parallel Approach* (Piavano, 2004), also known as the *Simultaneous Approach* (Chazan, 2003; Nilsson, 2006), which advocates that a sole therapist would conduct a treatment process with the parents – parallel to the treatment process of their child. This way of work is customary in care centres for children with autism in Israel, where I worked for ten years. But while the parents' counselling sessions being conducted in these care centres are verbally based, I have adjusted the body of knowledge known in music therapy for families of children with autism to meet the parents' daily needs, and developed a paradigm to incorporate music in different ways within the parents' counselling sessions conducted in the MOPC model.

The setting of the MOPC model is combined with counselling sessions for the parents, which occur twice a month focusing on the idea of 'music as a tool' (Malloch and Trevarthen, 2008), parallel to intensive individual music therapy sessions for the children, which occur twice a week. The intimate relationships that the therapist establishes with the child and with the parents allow the therapist to provide a treatment plan for the whole family, addressing the variable needs of the different members of the family.

The unique features of MOPC embrace the therapeutic understandings gathered through the clinical and research evidence in music therapy and autism, aiming to share and cooperate with the parents in order to facilitate everyday life through music. As a clinician, I follow the child's lead, a basic concept in music therapy with children (e.g. Wigram and Elefant, 2006; Holck, 2004; Holck, 2004; Wigram and Elefant, 2006), and in parent counselling strive to maintain the ability to follow their lead, in order to address and resonate with their changing needs. But following the parents' lead is not enough in order to achieve and maintain a collaborative relationship between the clinician and the parents. The craft of creating a relationship based on partnership with the parents, where parents are encouraged and empowered to explore and use their mental assets, is a prime goal within this model, and music takes a central role in this process. This corresponds with the 'Resource-Oriented Music Therapy' approach (Rolvsjord, 2010), which advocates perceiving each patient as a whole, focusing on the patient's strengths and resources parallel to his weaknesses, and highlight the continuous dialogue between the 'healthy parts' and the 'unhealthy parts' of each individual.

The population

The children

The American Psychiatric Association (2013) defines autism as a set of neurodevelopmental disorders that are diagnosed behaviourally and usually appear in early childhood and persist throughout life. The general characteristics of autism are impairments in social interaction and communication skills, integrated with restrictive, repetitive or stereotyped patterns of behaviour. Within the autism spectrum, a term first used by Wing (1995), a large variety of levels of individual abilities and wide clinical presentations are covered. The American Psychiatric Association (2013) defines three main levels of autism severity according to the amount of support needed: level 1 – requiring support; level 2 – requiring substantial support; level 3 – requiring very substantial support. This diversity and large variety of presentations within individuals affected with autism presents a big challenge for clinical diagnosis as well as for therapeutic intervention.

Throughout this chapter, I use the term 'autism' rather than 'autism spectrum disorder', as it represents the way I grasp and perceive the autism condition. Instead of using a somewhat negative expression as 'disorder', which can give the impression that something is broken in people who are diagnosed with autism that needs to be fixed and repaired, I chose to perceive autism as a neurodevelopmental condition, and acknowledge its multidimensional presentations in persons with autism.

The parents

Understanding parents of children with autism is a complex task, as what unites them as members of the same group is attached to their *children's diagnosis* and not to specific characteristics of their own personality or behaviour. Moreover, autism can affect individuals from all racial groups, socio-economic backgrounds and levels of intelligence (American Psychiatric Association, 2013), disqualifying any distribution of this population according to demographic characteristics. Nevertheless, literature in the field of social work and psychology argues that the diagnosis of the child within the autism spectrum has a powerful effect on the stress level of the parents. The literature concludes that the similar challenges which these parents need to cope with can be observed as unifying factors (Holroyd and McArthur, 1976; Baker-Ericzen et al., 2005; Pisula, 2007; Schieve et al., 2007).

Raising a child with autism is typically a challenging experience for parents; it begins early in the child's life, lasts throughout his or her development and growth, and is associated with a host of personal, familial and vocational problems (Whitman, 2004). These challenges include obtaining the initial diagnosis, finding appropriate treatment and intervention services, establishing appropriate parenting practices and coping with a substantial financial burden of paying for services. Many of these challenges are unique to the disability and are likely a consequence of attempting to cope with the communication deficits and restrictive behaviours associated with the autism spectrum (Jarbrink et al., 2003).

Parents who have children with autism endure a significant amount of stress (Abbeduto et al., 2004; Duarte et al., 2005; Konstantareas and Papageorggiou, 2006; Montes and Halterman, 2007). Studies show that they experience more stress, not only compared to parents of typically developed children, but also compared to parents of children with other developmental disabilities (Schieve et al., 2007). These findings raise a question as to whether autism functions as a source of stress for parents. i Significant research attempts to isolate the specific factors producing parenting stress and examine the relationship between child characteristics and daily functioning of mothers. Irritability, slowness, hyper-activity, communication and social interaction deficiencies were identified as stress elevators for mothers (Tomanik, Harris and Hawkins, 2004). Moreover, Davis and Carter (2008) found that children's deficit in social skills were predictive of par-enting stress for mothers of toddlers with autism. Also, increased level of behaviour problems (e.g. self-regulation difficulties and externalising behaviour) is significantly related to increase in parenting stress (Lecavalier, Leone and Wiltz, 2006; Davis and Carter, 2008).

Theoretical perspective

There is an increased awareness of the importance of a good parent–child relationship in the development of communication skills in both children with typical development (Edwards, 2011) and children with autism (Thompson, 2012). The goal in working with young children with autism has been underlined by Prizant, Wetherby and Rydell (2000) as giving the children the opportunity to experience ongoing social interactions with family members and friends as successful and emotionally fulfilling. A trusting and secure relationship is the fundamental element and the result of success in communication with others (Prizant et al., 2000, p. 218). Therefore, social, cognitive and communication development underpins trusting relationships with others who are emotionally attuned (Bruner, 1995; Prizant et al., 2000; Solomon et al., 2014). Supporting and influencing the child's motivation to stay engaged and excited about relationships is crucial for successful social development (Poulsen, Rodger and Ziviani, 2006; Campbell, Milbourne and Wilcox, 2008). Therefore, it is clear that the partners for interaction, whether parents, family members or friends, should be a part of this support system (Schertz and Odom, 2007; Thompson and McFerran, 2015; Gottfried, 2016; Gottfried et al., 2018; Wetherby et al., 2000). This ecological framework perceives the child's development in relation with the family's system of relationships (Winnicott, 1952; Bronfenbrenner, 1975).

The challenges of working therapeutically with parents have been described since the beginning of psychoanalytical theories, usually addressing it as a marginal supplement to the treatment process of children (Oren, 2012). Within developmental theory (Winnicott, 1964, 1971; Stern, 1985) and attachment theory (Bowlby, 1988) the work with parents takes a central role, as the parent–child dyad is seen as the core for an intact emotional development of the child. A full review of the history and different programmes available to work with parents is beyond the scope of this chapter. However, it is necessary to briefly acknowledge the basic theories which formed my understandings of parent–child relationships in general, and in families of autistic children in particular. The object relations theory, developed in the 1960s, presented the child's psychological development as connected with his or her parents and people around him. This theory perceives the primary relationship of the infant with his or her care figure (usually the mother) as the basis of his or her personality development as an adult (Mahler, 1965; Winnicott, 1971). Winnicott (1964) observed and understood infants from the perspective of the infant–mother dyad and interpreted the infants' behaviours and expressions within the context of early interactions between them and their mothers. He was an advocate of working closely with parents, consulting and supporting them, emphasising the idea of the relationship within the infant–mother dyad as significantly influencing the emotional–psychological development of the child. A central idea of his work was to empower mothers to provide a good mental holding and physical handling and become 'good-enough' mothers to their children (ibid). Attachment theory (Bowlby, 1988) emphasised the influence of the attachment in infancy on the future development of the child. Bowlby assumed that a baby is born with the ability to connect and with a congenital nature to seek connections. Infants need feedback of warmth, caring and closeness from their primary caregiver, in addition to their primary needs to be fed and to sleep. Both Bowlby (1988) and Winnicott (1967, 1971) hold the idea that an infant is not a separate entity but maintains a constant connection with his or her caregiver (usually the mother). Stern describes normal development as based on the essential 'self', meaning the development of self-identity in infancy (Stern, 2004). Like Winnicott, Stern emphasised the importance of mirroring as capturing the idea of the infant being understood by his or her parent, and the infant's expressions are meaningful to them.

At the core of autism are impairments in social and interaction skills (American Psychiatric Association, 2013), which might have a significant effect on the primary relationship between the infant and the parents. In contrast to traditional psychological perception of treatment, therapists who work with children with autism need to focus more on the quality of relationships living in the here-and-now, and put less attention on the past (Alvarez, 1999). The 'emptiness' that might be felt when interacting with an autistic child, is pinned to the numerous repetitions and 'resting-state' that a child with autism might exhibit. This calls for the interacting partners (whether they are parents, family members or therapists) to be 'live-company', and gently move on the continuum of closeness-remoteness with the child (Alvarez, 2002).

Parent counselling

One way of working with parents is through conducting parentcounselling sessions. The broad definition of parent counselling refers to any consultation between a professional and a parent (Guli, 2005). A narrower definition refers to parent counselling as a structured, problem-solving collaborative relationship between a consultant (e.g. counsellor, psychologist, therapist) and one or more parents (Holcomb-McCoy, 2009). As opposed to the 'conjoint behavioural consultation' (Sheridan, Kratochwill, and Bergan, 1996), which is an extension of behavioural consultation that was popular during the 1970s, the MOPC model stands in line with the *values- based parent counselling* (Nelson et al., 2000), which focuses on the family's values as the main aspect of counselling. In this paradigm, the consultant should abandon the role of the expert and value the knowledge that parents and community members bring to counselling sessions (Nelson et al., 2000), striving to create a partnership with the parents (Davis et al., 2002).

Following the growing understanding of the parents' role in their child's emotional development, two main therapeutic intervention models have been developed, treating both the needs of the child and the parent. The first therapeutic intervention, which stands also at the core of the MOPC model, is the simultaneous treatment (Chazan, 2003), known also as the parallel-treatment (Nilsson, 2006), which involves one therapist who treats separately, but in parallel, both child and parents. Within this model, the therapist strives to develop trust-worthy relationships, maintaining 'parallel-empathy' (Nilsson, 2006). This means that the therapist must must reflect on the transference and countertransference that the children and their parents evoke in her or him. This reflective process is complex, though essential in order to enable a trustworthy alliance with both parties involved in therapy.

The second therapeutic intervention is the dyadic model which involves one therapist who treats the child and the parents within the same sessions, putting the parent–child relationship at the focus of treatment (McDonough, 2000; Lieberman, 2004). The MOPC can also be practised within this model, in con-ducting parent counselling sessions parallel to the dyadic sessions. This will provide an opportunity for the parents to reflect on the mutual therapy session together with the music therapist, to deepen their understandings of what is going on between them and their child, and acknowledge the role that music takes within this relationship. These two models refer to an interpersonal inner layer, which represents inner processes of the ability to create change and develop as a parent. Working with parents on this level relies on formulating the parents' expectations, their needs, beliefs, ways of thinking and their ability to reflect, interpret and regulate emotions (Cohen, 2007).

Music therapy with parents of children with autism

Literature reveals two international approaches to work within music therapy with parents of children with autism (Edwards, 2011). The first is the international field of family-centred practice, especially work with infants and their parents in the early years. The second is based on the theoretical principles of communicative musicality (Malloch and Trevarthen, 2008), and knowledge of early musical skills and development (Trehub, 2003). The second approach aims to understand how and why musical interaction with a qualified music therapist can offer a potential pathway to resolving difficulties that are occurring in, or are a result of, the first relationship. Both of these theoretical frameworks demonstrate an increasing awareness within the music therapy field of the importance of successful attach-ment, and the rich possibilities of remediating unsuccessful attachment experiences through musical means within music therapy (Edwards, 2011).

Cooperating with parents of children with autism in music therapy is found in the literature since the 1970s. Some authors describe an approach of *teaching* parents how to interact with their child with autism using imitation, call and response and echo clapping (e.g. Benenzon, 1976). Others describe how *modeling* enables parents to use musical gestures during interactions with their child (e.g. Oldfield, 2006). Occasionally in these examples, the music therapist discusses progress of the child with the parents, emphasising his or her strengths.

In the past two decades, studies on the effect of music therapy with families of children with autism have expanded (Oldfield, 2006; Oldfield and Flower, 2008; Larsen, 2011; Thompson, 2012; Gottfried, 2016; Blauth, 2017), showing a greater interest among music therapists in this field. While some of these studies support the effectiveness of mutual music therapy sessions for children and their parents on improving their interaction through music-making, songs and musical improvisations (Oldfield, 2006; Oldfield and Flower, 2008; Larsen, 2011), other studies highlight the beneficial effect of parent counselling sessions, conducted parallel to music therapy sessions, on the parents' ability to identify their children's needs more clearly, and interact adequately with them, addressing their unique needs and strengths (Gottfried, 2016; Blauth, 2017). In all of these studies, it is shown that as a result of participating in music therapy sessions or participating in parent counselling sessions provided by a music therapist, parents were able to adopt certain musical interventions, and incorporate them in their interactions with their child.

MOPC research

Objective

The objective of this mixed-methods study was to investigate both the effect and experience of Music-Oriented Parent Counselling (MOPC) on the level of parental stress, quality of life perception and daily use of music in the home environment by parents of children with autism.

Methods

Linked to the international TIME-A RCT project, my Ph.D. study followed a fixed QUANT/QUAL triangulation mixed methods design. Thirteen participants were enrolled for a five months' intervention, randomly assigned to either 'minimal MOPC' (three sessions) or 'maximum MOPC' (ten sessions) and 'with music therapy for the child' or 'without music therapy' in 2×2 groups. Data was analysed using the following quantitative measurement tools: Questionnaire for Resources and Stress (QRS; Friedrich et al. 1983), Quality of Life VAS (QoL; EuroQoL Group, 1990), Music in Everyday Life questionnaire[1] (MEL; Gottfried & Thompson, unpublished) all conducted at baseline and at the end of intervention. Qualitative analysis focused on semi-structured interviews, conducted with all the participants at the end of intervention.

Results

For the first outcome measure – *Level of Stress*: Quantitative results showed that level of stress did not increase, but no significant improvement occurred in any of the groups. The qualitative findings, however, revealed that parents gained new understandings of their child's situation as well as practical tools to cope, most of them identifiedmusical tools, which lowered their stress level.

For the second outcome measure – *Quality of Life*: Quantitative results showed that QoL of the parents improved, although not significantly, among parents who participated in 10 MOPC sessions compared to three MOPC sessions ($p = .123$); Change in parents' perception of their child's QoL was significantly greater in families whose children participated in music therapy sessions ($p = .011$). Qualitative findings identified Quality of Life as a complex term, not influenced directly by MOPC sessions.

For the third outcome measure – *Music in Everyday Life*: Quantitative results showed a significant change in the use of music in routine activities among parents who participated in ten MOPC sessions compared to those who participated in three MOPC sessions ($p = .020$). The change in the use of music in joint activities was larger, although non-significant, among families whose children participated in music therapy sessions compared to those who didn't receive music therapy session ($p = .123$). Qualitative findings showed that parents of all groups implemented ideas and musical tools they had gained during sessions and expanded their use of music with their children.

Additional findings of the qualitative analysis resulted in three main themes that emerged from the interviews with parents : Learning Experience, Enabling Space and Music in everyday life. These themes capture the essence of the Music-Oriented Parent Counselling process, where music in everyday life is the core of the process, developing through a learning experience, which can occur within an enabling relationship between the music therapist counsellor and the parents (Figure 2.1).

MOPC – Clinical approach

Parent counselling sessions

Music-Oriented Parent Counselling (MOPC) is fuelled by the strong sense of committment I feel after working for so many years in music therapy with children with autism and their parents. As much as I have seen miracles happen when music has become the ultimate bridge between me and the children in music therapy, I have felt it is my responsibility to facilitate the parents' understanding of the role of music in their children's lives, and make music accessible for them. It stands in line with my worldview of perceiving the relationship between the parents and myself as equal and collaborative, as opposed to perceiving myself as the expert and the parents as the help seekers. This relationship combines the parents' priceless knowledge of their child with my professional experience and knowledge, which evolves over time. A central motive within this model is the use of music and music-therapy techniques during parents' sessions; music-making and music-listening have two goals: (1) to foster the parents' reflexivity concerning daily situations, dilemmas and empowerment through the experience of music; (2) to

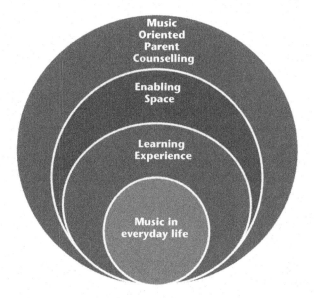

FIGURE 2.1 Representation of the parents' overall experience of MOPC, as revealed from the qualitative analysis

present the concept of 'music as a tool', and offer the parents the opportunity to practice and adopt certain musical activities that they can integrate into their daily interactions with their child.

MOPC involves supportive conversations for parents about current difficulties and concerns arising from their child's diagnosis. Music is central to the sessions, and parents are invited to share musical compositions of their own choice, which represent their feeling in the 'here-and-now'. After listening to the musical piece together, a discussion takes place on the meaning and the context of their choice of music. Parents are invited to improvise with musical instruments during the counselling sessions, to allow a non-verbal way of exploring their feelings, thoughts, worries, aspirations and hopes. A conversation follows each improvisation, aimed at encouraging parents to make connections between the musical experience and their lives. As an overarching principle, this model considers the child's needs and capabilities alongside the parents' strengths and challenges. This may be an opprtunity forthe parents to consider their own needs, which they may have neglected while being preoccupied with their child's needs. As the MOPC research showed, parents stated that the most striking and valuable thing they gained from the process is perceiving music as a tool and using it during difficult periods during the day to foster a meaningful engagement with their children.

Music therapy approach with the children

The music therapy approach applied in this model is based on findings from previous music therapy research (e.g. Edgerton, 1994; Holck, 2004; Kim et al., 2009) and developmental psychology (Stern, 2010), a psychodynamic approach and improvisational techniques (Geretsegger et al., 2012). Generally, the music therapy sessions should include both structured activities and child-led parts and consist of active music making by the therapist and the child, and verbal comments. In musical terms, this may involve matching, sustaining, or complementing 'musical' features of the child's behaviour (pulse, rhythmic pattern, dynamic or melodic contour, timbre; Geretsegger et al., 2015), thus creating moments of synchronisation and 'meeting' (cf. Schumacher and Calvet-Crupa, 1999; Kim et al., 2009). It also uses therapeutic principles fundamental to music therapy with children with autism, such as fostering emotional expression, being emotionally involved in music, engaging the client in musical interaction and encouraging vocalisation.

The role of the music therapist

A music therapist following the MOPC model needs to be experienced in working both with children with autism and their parents, and have a significant knowledge of the difficulties these parents are facing in daily life. One of the greatest challenges for the music therapist in this model is to act and intervene according to the needs of the child AND his or her parents; the music therapist needs to be able to 'hold in her/his mind' both parts of the treatment, and be aware of his or her own feelings that arise during the process. The focus of the feelings might change during the therapeutic process, sometimes be in identification with the child, sometimes with the parents and sometimes with both (Nilsson, 2006). It is also important that the music therapist be aware of his or her advanced musical skills and create a comfortable atmosphere for parents to experience the musicality within themselves. In my experience, parents tend to hesitate whenever I propose we play music during sessions. Music–making may be unfamiliar to them, and even when they are interested they initially may refuse or avoid playing, explaining this by not knowing *how* to play musical instruments', or not playing well enough. It might be also that perceiving me as a skilled musician inhibits their willingness to explore. As many of the parents have shared with me, there is a big difference between loving to listen to music and actually playing it. I then contextualize the use of music as an expressive tool, that helps them to explore their own feelings or to communicate with their child.

Another aim of the music therapist in this model is to create a bridge between the relationship built with the child and the relationships formed with the parents. This involves forming a professional judgement as to when and to what extent to offer advice on parenting. For example: if the therapist observes during music therapy sessions that the child responds positively to singing, engages better and succeeds in maintaining contact for longer periods of time, he or she may want to recommend that the parents sing with their child, so they can experience the same things the music therapist has experienced in therapy. It is most important to describe this to the parents in a way that won't evoke anxiety or feelings of incompetency as to *their* ability to sing to their child. In situations in which singing is somewhat 'foreign' to the parents, and does not come naturally and freely, such a recommendation might evoke feelings of being 'not-good-enough parents' when it comes to engagingwith their child. The music therapist must then explore together with the parents the specific use of music that suits their capabilities and the type of musical activity that would come naturally to them. The MEL assessment (Gottfried et al., 2018) can be an excellent tool to collect information about the spontaneous ways that parents use music with their children. This will highlight what comes naturally to the parents, and be useful in planning the treatment programme for the family.

It is my experience as a supervisor that sometimes music therapists conceive of working with parents as an onerous task which they are requested to deal with and don't feel knowledgeable enough to succeed in it. These feelings are certainly authentic, as working with families is taught very briefly in most music therapy training programmes, and CPD courses in this area are rare. Often, supervision by an expert in the field is the only available support. Feeling ill-equipped might have a significant effect on the relationship being formed between the music therapist and the parents, and supervision is key. The creation of a safe therapeutic place is just as important for the parents as it is for the children in order to be able to express themselves and gain trust in their relationship with us. Acceptance and a non-judgemental attitude are required. i According to Rustin's psychoanalytic approach (2000), it is useful for parents to be treated by child therapist who has an understanding of parent have hasundergone 'working with parents' training, since this allows dedicating more attention to the impact of the patient's internal difficulties on parental functioning and to the projective identifications within family relationships.

Vignette

Dana contacted my private music therapy clinicabout music therapy treatment for her son Michael. She and her husband loved music, and Dana thought music therapy sessions would have a positive influence on Michael. Dana felt that Michael was not developing well but was told by her doctor to 'give him time' to progress. At the age of 20 months, Michael was diagnosed with autism, and by the time he was referred to me, the diagnosis was changed to 'severe autism'. Michael was a very handsome six-year-old boy, non-verbal, very restless, was seeking non-stop tactile stimulation and could barely focus on one thing for more than ten seconds. When I first met Dana, she looked sad and worried; her parenting experience had been very tiring and desperate, far from what she had imagined and expected. It seemed as if she was walking on unstable ground, looking for help and guidance. Dana hoped that music therapy would help calm Michael, give him peace and even bring back the mutual enjoyment they once shared through music.

Ever since Michael was born, Dana used to sing to him Israeli children's songs. She used to put him on her lap, make loving eye contact and sing one song after another. As a baby, Michael had used to meet her gaze, smile and be restful. Dana had treasured these moments, and her eyes sparkled when she talked about them during counselling sessions. These moments of connection now seemed distant to her, as it was hard to capture Michael's attention for more than a few seconds, and even then, his attention was very fragile and could be interrupted easily.

I worked with Michael in music therapy twice a week, in parallel to the parent counselling sessions with his mother. Michael loved coming to the room and was constantly smiling. He was very restless, running from one side of the room to the other and had a hard time to maintain sensory regulation. Michael was very curious about any music that I produced; whether it was improvising on musical instruments, playing familiar songs or listening to music together – Michael would stop running around, and looked right at me. Whenever I used my voice in singing or in 'melodic speaking', Michael would move closer to me, make eye contact, and move his body from side to side. It was clear that he felt comfortable with the language of music and was drawn to it. Although not verbal, he used his voice freely. He mumbled, made sounds that resembled words, he talked in his own language.

In one session, Michael was talking in his personal language a lot. He made eye contact with me, and talked and talked. I started answering him in his own 'words', imitating but adding more musicality to them, organising my phrases with a steady beat I played on the drum. Soon, we had a whole 'conversation', in which Michael said a sentence and I answered him. This 'conversation' lasted throughout the session, and we engaged happily with each other. Michael looked as if it was the first time that someone understood him and interacted with him in his own language. This became our routine and Michael's musical language was present in every music therapy session we had.

At that time, parallel sessions with Dana continued and Dana kept expressing despair about her inability to capture Michael's attention and engage with him. Given my musical experiences with Michael, I encouraged Dana to share her relationship with music with me, so I could assess what came naturally to her in terms of using music. If Dana could feel comfortable using music, then music could become the bridge that would lead her back to her son. Dana gladly shared her childhood and more current experiences with music, emphasising her strong wish to incorporate music in her life as a mother. I reminded Dana of her story about singing children's songs to Michael when he was a baby, and asked her why she stopped. She reflected on my questions and answered that since receiving Michael's diagnosis, she had been unable to sing to him. 'But now', she said, 'as we had our second child, I started singing again to the "new" baby'. I asked Dana to express what music symbolises for her; she responded that for her, music symbolises life, happiness and hope. I carefully shared with Dana my understanding of the situation: after the diagnosis, there was no longer room for these things, and consequently, music could no longer exist between her and Michael. Now, with the new baby, there was a new opportunity to restore these qualities, so music wasalive again. I then shared with Dana the positive effect that singing and mumbling in Michael's invented language had on him. I emphasised that life, happiness and hope still there in him, and that her ability to use singing freely could help her meet Michael in his own musical world.

After six months of music therapy and parallel parent counselling sessions, Dana could find the music inside her again and incorporated singing in her interaction with Michael. By being a role model without taking over the relationship with Michael, I acted as a facilitator for a better relationship between Dana and her son. In this case, I used music in two ways: (1) as an experience in which the mother could express her feelings and gain deep insights; and (2) as a tool for the mother to engage and interact with her son. Although everyday life continues to have its difficulties and hardships, Dana feels more capable and empowered to deal with complex situations with Michael, and both of them experience meaningful moments of engagement and connection.

Discussion

Clinical practice of music therapists around the world who work regularly with children with autism is developing, where child-centred focus has gradually transferred to family-centred focus, emphasising the growing understandings of the importance of the parents' role in their children wellbeing. Also, music therapists are united by the wish to share their insights with parents, in order to help them communicate better with their children, and to hopefully relieve them of some of theirstress and feelings of ineptitude (Oldfield, 1993, 2006; Blauth 2017; Bull, 2008; Loth, 2008; Oldfield and Flower, 2008; Thompson, 2012; Gottfried, 2016). The MOPC model uses the parallel-treatment paradigm (Piavano, 2004), also known as the simultaneous-treatment (Chazan, 2003; Nilsson, 2006) paradigm, emphasising the role of a sole therapist who conducts therapy for the child and for the parents separately but parallel in time. In my experience, conducting separate and ongoing parent counselling sessions alongside the music therapy sessions of their child contributes greatly to the parents' ability to understand their child's needs, to acknowledge their own strengths and challenges, and to improve communication within the family. The counselling approach in MOPC seeks to form a partnership between the music therapist and the parents, combining the expertise and knowledge of the partners towards achieving shared goals, with mutual respect and collaboration.

Final thoughts and further recommendations

A lack of interaction skills and limited emotional expression are at the core of autism disorder. Daily life can be challenging for the whole family with a child with autism. Research evidences a high level of stress, especially in mothers, due to the need to provide their children with the suitable treatment and establish appropriate parenting practices. This model is based on the concept that music therapy offers more 'natural' and vital ways of interacting through music making. However, unlike other models in the field (Oldfield and Flower, 2008; Larsen,

2011; Thompson, 2012), this approach lacks the opportunity to provide *modelling* to the parents, as they are not a part of the music therapy sessions with their child, and therefore don't see the music therapist 'in action'. For some parents, this may pose a barrier to grasping the essence of the musical interaction. However, the ongoing counselling sessions with the same music therapist that treats their child allow the parents time to reflect, wonder, learn and develop as parents in relation to their child with autism.

Parents have described this model as a beneficial 'learning process' and as an 'enabling space', which has helped them to feel less stressed and more competent with their children with autism. Furthermore, parents have emphasised that music takes a central role within this model, and that the opportunities of 'music as a tool' were an exciting revelation to them.[2]

Notes

1 *The Music in Everyday Life (MEL) assessment was developed especially for the study; publication on reliability appeared in JMT* (Gottfried et al., 2018).
2 Further information on MOPC training opportunities can be directed to Dr Tali Gottfried: taligott@bezeqint.net

References

Abbeduto, L., Mailick Seltzer, M., Shattuck, P., Wyngaarden Krauss, M., Orsmond, G., and Murphy, M.M. (2004) 'Psychological well-being and coping in mothers of youth with autism, down syndrome or Fragile X syndrome', *American Journal on Mental Retardation*, 109(3), pp. 237–254.

Alvarez, A. (1999) 'Addressing the deficit: Developmentally informed psychotherapy with passive, "undrawn" children' in Alvarez, A., and Reid, S. (eds.) *Autism and personality: Findings from the Tavistock Autism Workshop*. London and New York: Routledge Publishers, pp. 49–61.

Alvarez, A. (2002) *Live company*. New York: Brunner-Routledge.

American Psychiatric Association. (2013) *Diagnostic and statistical manual of mental disorders*. 5th edn. Washington, DC: American Psychiatric Association.

Baker-Ericzen, M.J., Brookman-Frazee, L., and Stahmer, A. (2005) 'Stress levels and adaptability in parents of toddlers with and without autism spectrum disorders', *Research and Practice for Persons with Severe Disabilities*, 30, pp. 194–204.

Baron-Cohen, S. (2001) 'Theory of mind and autism: A review', *International Review of Research in Mental Retardation*, 23, pp. 169–205.

Benenzon, R.O. (1976) 'Music therapy in infantile autism', *British Journal of Music Therapy*, 7, pp. 10–17.

Blauth, L. (2017) 'Improving mental health in families with autistic children: Benefits of using video feedback in parent counselling sessions offered alongside music therapy', *Health Psychology Report*, 5(2), pp. 1–13.

Bowlby, J. (1988) *A secure base: Clinical application of attachment theory*. London: Routledge.

Bronfenbrenner, U. (1975) 'Is early intervention effective?' in Freidlander, B., Sterritt, G., and Kirk, G. (eds.) *Exceptional infant: Assessment and intervention* (vol. 3). New York: Brunner/Mazel, pp. 449–475.

Bruner, J. (1995) 'From joint attention to the meeting of minds: An introduction' in Moore, C., and Dunham, P.J. (eds.) *Joint attention: Its origins and role in development*. New Jersey: Lawrence Erlbaum Associates, pp. 1–14.

Bull, R. (2008) 'Autism and the family: Group music therapy with mothers and children' in Oldfield, A., and Flower, C. (eds.) *Music therapy with children and their families*. London: Jessica Kingsley Publishers, pp. 71–88.

Campbell, P.H., Milbourne, S., and Wilcox, M.J. (2008) 'Adaptation interventions to promote participation in natural settings', *Infants & Young Children*, 21(2), p. 94.

Chazan, S.E. (2003) *Simultaneous treatment of parent and child*. London: Jessican Kingsley Publishers,.

Cohen, A. (2007) *The parenting experience: Relationships, coping and development*. Jerusalem: Ach Publications.

Davis, N.O., and Carter, A.S. (2008) 'Parenting stress in mothers and fathers of toddlers with autism spectrum disorders: Associations with child characteristics. *Journal of Autism and Developmental Disorders*, 38, pp. 1278–1291.

Davis, H., Day, C., and Bidmead, C. (2002) *Working in partnership with parents: The parent adviser model*. London: Harcourt Assessment.

Duarte, C.S., Bordin, I.A., Yazigi, L., and Monny, J. (2005) 'Factors associated with stress in mothers of children with autism', *Journal of Learning Disabilities*, 9(4), pp. 416–427.

Edgerton, C.L. (1994) 'The effect of improvisational music therapy on the communication behaviours of autistic children', *Journal of Music Therapy*, 31(1), pp. 31–61.

Edwards, J. (2011) The use of music therapy to promote attachment between parents and infants. *Arts Psychotherapy*, 38, pp. 190–195.

EuroQoL Group. (1990) 'A new facility for the measurement of health-related quality of life', *Health Policy*, 16(3), 199–208.

Friedrich, W. N., Greenberg, M. T., and Crnick, K. (1983) 'Short form of the questionnaire on resources and stress', *American Journal of Mental Deficiency*, 88, 41–48.

Geretsegger, M., Holck, U., and Gold, C. (2012) 'Randomized controlled trial of improvisational music therapy's effectiveness for children with autism spectrum disorders (TIME-A): Study protocol', *BMC Pediatrics*, 12, 2. doi: 10.1186/1471-2431-12-2.

Gertesegger, M., Elefant, C., Mossler, K.A., and Gold, C. (2014) 'Music therapy for people with autism spectrum disorder (review)', *Cochrane Library*, 6, pp. 1–64.

Geretsegger, M., Holck, U., Elefant, C., and Gold, C. (2015) 'Common characteristics of improvisational approaches in music therapy for children with autism spectrum disorder: Developing treatment guidelines', *Journal of Music Therapy*, 52(2), 258–281. https://doi.org/10.1093/jmt/thv005

Gottfried, T. (2016) 'Music-oriented counselling model for parents of children with autism spectrum disorder' in Lindhal-Jacobsen, S., and Thompson, G. (eds.) *Music therapy with families: Therapeutic Approaches and theoretical perspectives*. London and Philadelphia: Jessica Kingsley Publishers, pp. 116–134.

Gottfried, T., Thompson, G., Elefant, C., and Gold, C. (2018) 'Reliability of the music in everyday life (MEL) scale: A parent-report assessment for parents of children on the autism spectrum' *Journal of Music Therapy*, 55(2), pp. 133–155.

Guli, L.A. (2005) Evidence-based parent consultation with school-related outcomes. *School Psychology* Quarterly, 20, pp. 455–472.

Holck, U. (2004) 'Turn-taking in music therapy with children with communication disorders', *British Journal of Music Therapy* 18(2), pp. 45–54.

Holcomb-McCoy, C. (2009) *Cultural considerations in parent consultation (ACAPD-25)*. Alexandira, VA: American Counselling Association.

Holroyd, J., and McArthur, D. (1976) 'Mental retardation and stress on the parents: A contrast between down's syndrome and childhood autism', *American Journal of Mental Deficiency*, 80, pp. 431–436.

Jarbrink, K., Fombonne, E., and Knapp, M. (2003) 'Measuring the parental, service and cost impacts of children with autistic spectrum disorder: A pilot study', *Journal of Autism and Developmental Disorders*, 33(4), pp. 395–402.

Kim, J., Wigram, T., and Gold, C. (2009) 'Emotional, motivational and interpersonal responsiveness of children with autism in improvisational music therapy', *Autism* 13(4), pp. 389–409.

Konstantareas, M.M., and Papageorggiou, V. (2006) 'Effects of temperament, symptom severity and level of functioning on maternal stress in Greek children and youth with ASD', *Autism* 10(6), pp. 593–607.

Larsen, A.R. (2011) *Musikterapeutisk Vejledning* (English abstract). Unpublished Master's Thesis Aalborg University, DK.

Lecavalier, L., Leone, S., and Wiltz, J. (2006) 'The impact of behaviour problems on caregiver stress in young people with autism spectrum disorders', *Journal of Intellectual Disability Research*, 50, pp. 172–183.

Lieberman, F.E. (2004) 'Child–parent psychotherapy, A relationship based approach to the treatment of mental health disorders in infancy and early childhood' in Sameroff, A.J., McDonough, S.C., and Rosenblum, K.L. (eds.) *Treating parent–infant relationship problems*. New York: Guilford Press, pp. 97–122.

Loth, H. (2008) 'Music therapy groups for families with a learning-disabled toddler: Bridging some gaps' in Oldfield, A., and Flower, C. (eds.) *Music therapy with children and their families*. London: Jessica Kingsley Publishers, pp. 53–70.

Mahler, M.S. (1965) 'On the significance of the normal separation-individuation phase' in Schur, M. (ed.) *Drives, affects and behaviour* (vol. 2). New York: International Universities Press.

Malloch, S., and Trevarthen, C. (2008) *Communicative musicality: Exploring the basis of human companionship*. Oxford: Oxford University Press.

McDonough, S.C. (2000) 'Interaction guidance: An approach for difficult to engage families' in Zeanah, C. (ed.) *Handbook of infant mental health*. New York: Guildford Press, pp. 485–493.

Montes, G., and Halterman, J.S. (2007) 'Psychological functioning and coping among mothers of children with autism: A population-based study', *Pediatrics*, 119(5), pp. 1040–1046.

Moore, T. (2009) 'The nature and significance of relationships in the lives of children with and without developmental disabilities', paper presented at the National Conference of the Early Intervention Association of Aotearoa, Auckland, New Zealand, 30 March-1 April 2009.

Nelson, G., Amio, J.L., Prilleltensky, I., and Nickels, P. (2000) 'Partnerships for implementing school and community prevention programs', *Journal of Educational and Psychological* Consultation, 11, pp. 121–145.

Nilsson, M. (2006) 'To be the sole therapist: Children and parents in simultaneous psychotherapy', *Journal of Infant, Child & Adolescent Psychotherapy*, 5(2), pp. 206–225.

Oldfield, A. (1993) 'Music therapy with families' in Wigram, T., and Heal, M. (eds.) *Music therapy in health and education*. London: Jessica Kingsley Publishers, pp. 46–54.

Oldfield, A. (2006) *Interactive music therapy: A positive approach.* London: Jessica Kingsley Publishers.

Oldfield, A. (2011) 'Parents' perceptions of being in music therapy sessions with their children: What is our role as therapists with parents?' in Edwards, J. (ed.) *Music therapy and parent–infant bonding.* Oxford: Oxford University Press, pp. 58–72.

Oldfield, A., and Flower, C. (2008) *Music therapy with children and their families.* London: Jessica Kingsley Publishers.

Oren, D. (2012) 'An optional concept for therapeutic work with parents and parenthood: Psychodynamic parenthood therapy', *Clinical Child Psychology and* Psychiatry, 4, pp. 553–570.

Piavano, B. (2004) 'Parenthood and parental functions as a result of the experience of parallel psychotherapy with children and parents', *International Forum of Psychoanalysis,* 13, pp. 187–200.

Pisula, E. (2007) 'A comparative study of stress profiles in mothers of children with Autism and those of children with Down's Syndrome'. *Journal of Applied Research in Intellectual Disabilities,* 20, pp. 274–278.

Poulsen, A., Rodger, S., and Ziviani, J.M. (2006) 'Understanding children's motivation from a self-determination theoretical perspective: Implications for practice', *Australian Occupational Therapy Journal,* 53(2), pp. 78–86.

Prizant, B., Wetherby, A., and Rydell, P. (2000) 'Communication intervention issues for children with autism spectrum disorders' in Wetherby, A.M., and Prizant, B.M. (eds.) *Autism spectrum disorders: A transactional developmental perspective* (vol. 9). Baltimore: Paul H Brookes Publishing, pp. 193–224.

Rolvsjord, R. (2010) *Resource-oriented music therapy in mental health care.* Gilsum, NH: Barcelona Publishers.

Rustin, M. (2000) 'Dialogues with parents' in Rustin, M. (ed.) *Work with parents: psycho-analytic psychotherapy with children and adolescents.* London: Karnack Books.

Schertz, H.H., and Odom, S.L. (2007) 'Promoting joint attention in toddlers with autism: a parent-mediated developmental model', *Journal of Autism and Developmental Disorders,* 37, pp. 1562–1575.

Schieve, L.A., Blumberg, S.J., Rice, C., Visser, S.N., and Boyle, C. (2007) 'The re-lationship between autism and parenting stress', *Pediatrics,* 119 (Suppl. 1), pp. 114–121.

Schumacher, K., and Calvet-Crupa, C. (1999) 'The "AQR" – an analysis system to evaluate the quality of relationship during music therapy', *Nordic Journal of Music Therapy,* 8(2), pp. 188–191.

Sheridan, S.M., Kratochwill, T.R., and Bergan, J.R. (1996) *Conjoint behavioural consultation: A procedural manual.* New York: Plenum Press.

Solomon, R., Van Egeren, L., Mahoney, G., Quon Huber, M., and Zimmerman, P. (2014) 'PLAY Project home consultation intervention program for young children with autism spectrum disorder: A randomized controlled trial', *Journal of Developmental & Behavioral Pediatrics,* 35(8), pp. 475–485.

Stern, D. (2010) *Forms of vitality.* Oxford: Oxford University Press.

Stern, D.N. (1985) *The interpersonal world of the infant: A view from psychoanalysis and devel-opmental psychology.* New York: Basic Books.

Stern, D.N. (2004) 'The motherhood constellation: Therapeutic approaches to early relational problems' in McDonough, C.S., Rosenblum, K.L., and Sameroff, A.J. (eds.) *Treating parent-infant relationship problems: Strategies for intervention.* New York: Guilford press, pp. 29–42.

Thompson, G. (2012) 'Family-centered music therapy in the home environment: pro-moting interpersonal engagement between children with autism spectrum disorder and their parents', *Music Therapy Perspectives,* 30(2), pp. 109–116.

Thompson, G., and McFerran, K. (2015) '"We've got a special connection": Qualitative analysis of descriptions of change in the parent–child relationship by mothers of young children with autism spectrum disorder', *Nordic Journal of Music Therapy,* 24(1), pp. 3–26.

Tomanik, S., Harris, G.E., and Hawkins, J. (2004) 'The relationship between behaviours exhibited by children with autism and maternal stress', *Journal of Intellectual & Developmental Disability,* 29, pp. 16–26.

Trehub, S.E. (2003) 'The developmental origins of musicality', *Nature Neuroscience,* 6, pp. 669–673.

Wetherby, A.M., Prizant, B.M., and Schuler, A.L. (2000) 'Understanding the nature of communication and language impairments' in Wetherby, A.M., and Prizant, B.M. (eds.) *Autism spectrum disorders: A transactional developmental perspective* (vol. 9). Baltimore: Paul H Brookes Publishing, pp. 109–141.

Whitman, T.L. (2004). *The development of autism: A self-regulatory perspective.* London: Jessica Kingsley.

Wigram, T., and Elefant, C. (2006). 'Therapeutic dialogues in music: Nurturing musicality of communication in children with autistic spectrum disorder and Rett syndrome' in Trevarthern, C., and Malloch, S. (eds.) *Communicative musicality.* Oxford: OUP, pp. 423–445.

Winnicott, D.W. (1952) *Through paediatrics to psychoanalysis: Collected papers.* London: Karnac.

Wing, L. (1995) *Autistic spectrum disorders: An aid to diagnosis.* England, UK: The National Autistic Society.

Wing, L. (1988) 'The continuum of autistic characteristics' in Schopler, E., and Mesibov, G. (eds.) *Diagnosis and assessment in autism.* Boston: Springer, pp. 91–110.

Winnicott, D.W. (1964) *The child, the family and the outside world.* England: Penguin Books.

Winnicott, D.W. (1971) *Playing and reality* 1st Ed. London: Tavistock Publications.

Winnicott, D.W. (1986) *Playing and reality.* London: Pelican.

3

'WHAT ARE THESE IRRUPTIONS OF THE SPIRIT?' EXPLORING (THE ELUSIVE) THERAPEUTIC PROPERTIES OF PUPPETRY AND PUPPET-CRAFT WITHIN DRAMATHERAPY CLINICAL PRACTICE WITH YOUNG PEOPLE

Daniel Stolfi

Introduction

In the summer of 2012, I was in Utah conducting research into aspects of mental health among Native American communities of the southwestern United States and had been invited to attend a residential programme for at risk Native American teenagers in the area. While my involvement with the youth pro-gramme did not include any hands-on work with puppetry, it afforded me a unique opportunity to explore some of the remarkable rock art in the area. The region has some of the richest concentrations of petroglyph and pictograph sites in the United States and is archaeological evidence of the ancestral presence of many of today's contemporary Native American communities, as well as a reminder of their deeply embedded affinity with the land.

Be that as it may, of the many influences and sources from which I draw inspiration for my puppetry work with young people, prehistoric rock art remains one of the most suggestive and most indelible, above all, because of the uni-versality of its aesthetic and symbolic characteristics – that is, the rudimentary, childlike drawings, the relational and cohering energy contained in the fragility of the etchings and markings, the rugged solidity of its primary material, its elusive embeddedness and the fascination and allure of its anonymity, to mention just a few of its surprising qualities and characteristics. It has also had a profound in-fluence on shaping my theoretical thinking about the historicity, spatiality, ma-teriality, as well as the spiritual and ethical dimensions of creativity and creative expression – not least because it is also one of the first manifestations of human creative expression for which we have a record.

During my time in Utah, I was extremely fortunate to visit the Newspaper Rock State Historic Monument located near the Four Corners area of the country. Newspaper Rock, as it is commonly known, is a bulging mass of sandstone on which a large panel of petroglyphs and other etchings have been scratched over the centuries. It is probably the most visited prehistoric rock art site in the region, and like many other similar sites, it is remote and out of the way. On the day in question, however, I was the only visitor at the site and was enveloped by the overarching silence of that vast landscape.

In Navajo, the rock is called 'Tse' Hane' (rock that tells a story).[1] The panel itself is roughly 20 square metres in dimension and framed by a huge outcropping of rock reminiscent of a proscenium arch, creating for the viewer the sensation of standing before a shadow-puppet theatre stage, witnessing a remarkable performance of timeless and otherworldly proportions. The constellation of humanoid and other figures, cartoon-like animals, six-toed footprints, symbols, initials, dates, geometric marks and scratches on the plane's surface telescopes at the same time it mirrors back to one the ambiguities of itself. It presents an impressive and unique tapestry of spatial, temporal and material textures and narratives in a huge aesthetic swathe. Ultimately, this 'rock that tells a story' is speaking to us about ourselves in one of our most basic creative idioms, telling us the unfinished story-within-a-story about the perpetual re-enactment of self in relation to other and, undoubtedly, in celebration of life in some of its many and nuanced manifestations.

Essentially, it is this fundamental dialogical element, polyvocality and sense of agency that I try to carry over into my creative and therapeutic thinking when I work with puppetry in both creative and therapeutic settings.

I believe that in the context of dramatherapy, creativity or creative expression is the client's most important resource – that it is the primary healing agent or catalyst in the client's therapeutic process. Moreover, it is both the fact and the manner that dramatherapy stimulates, harnesses and contains the client's creativity that sets it apart from the other psychotherapies. Therefore, it behoves the dramatherapist, first and foremost, to ensure their clients can have access to, use, and optimise this essential resource as much as possible in terms of its full range and all its properties and repertoires – that is, the symbolic, the aesthetic, the material, the technical, the subjective, the cultural and the ethical.

As far as the puppet (or object) itself is concerned, the underlying premise with which I am concerned is two-fold. Firstly, in dramatic terms, the puppet is simultaneously an elusive and contradictory yet embodied phenomenon in that it is co-constitutive of the liminal and dramatic space it inhabits. It exists as an inanimate object that is brought to life through human manipulation, while, on the other hand, it is simultaneously a subject and an object and, in my view, with its own complex agentic properties that allows it to straddle both these interconnected realms neutrally and comfortably – and sometimes anomalously, and sometimes subversively as well.

Secondly, in specifically therapeutic terms, the puppet is a dissociative and projective medium used for an integrative function. In one sense, the puppet has preserved its identity and legacy as a symbolic object used in sacred and ceremonial ritual practices and animistic belief systems dating back to the Pleistocene age. Meanwhile, it has also kept some of the numinous, revelatory, transformational and curative properties of those healing systems (Jurkowski, 2000; Wolff, 2000; Blumenthal, 2005; Stolfi, 2008, 2011). In contemporary clinical settings, it can become a versatile and highly sophisticated mechanism – primarily as a projective and embodied dramatic metaphor that lends itself to a wide range of applications for both children and adults. Used in this manner, its dynamic and unifying properties not only contain ambiguity, they establish coherence and continuity and can be regenerative and produce new value and new meaning.

Within this frame, therefore, I contend that the extent to which the client engages with the puppetry medium through the construction process (which may or may not include animating the object) is central to the therapeutic merits of using puppetry in dramatherapy settings. In making the puppet physically and materially, clients discover and build for themselves coherence and meaning. For this reason, the craft and the making of the object is more than indispensable, it is the most transformative and empowering part of the experience for the client and therefore probably the most important and most comprehensible facet of the therapeutic process for them. How the dramatherapist facilitates this accessibility for their clients is also a central and fundamental component of the enterprise and is essential to determining the nature of the therapeutic relationship in all its aspects.

The not, not here: the puppet as orphan

Dramatherapists need to foreground a more arts-based practice approach whereby it is the art form and the art practice itself that is the therapeutic catalyst and evidence rather than aspiring or conforming to over-determined empirically grounded medical explanatory models. Moreover, it should be a praxis that is inspired by a sensibility that is more interdisciplinary and more multi-modal and integrative – one that is more socio-culturally sensitive, inquisitive, invested in greater diversity and capable of accommodating the co-existence and mutuality of many platforms and many therapeutic issues, differences and populations. And, therefore, more tolerant and accepting of ambiguity, otherness, and uncertainty.

In my capacity as a therapist, artist and social scientist, I champion the therapeutic uses puppetry as a particular model of such praxis, and I would like to turn my attention now to consider a more theoretical discussion of the 'technology' of the medium and how I understand it in the context of the therapeutic setting under consideration. I am particularly interested in engaging with the spatiality and materiality of the puppet as a primary therapeutic constellation, and in exploring the puppet as a being and an entity that is also a highly integrated configuration full of complexity, offset by binary opposites, considerable nonlinearity, and with its own unique agency constituted through the visual, the sonic, the verbal and so forth.

As my starting point, I argue that the puppet is simultaneously both subject and object (a being and an entity) and therefore embodies and manifests both intersubjective and 'interobjective' (Morton, 2013) traits and properties. It can exist both as a character within a story (or a character that is the story) and as a physical and material object that is an aggregation of its parts over and above its 'situatedness' within any given narrative context or, even, its 'authoring' of such contexts. Moreover, character and object are co-constituted and co-exist through a process of symbolic synthesis and configuration that mimics (or is used therapeutically to mimic in some capacity – that is, through imitation, replication and role playing) and therefore aligns and connects the intersubjectivities of the client's self-process and individuation (Jung, 1940).

It is, therefore, worth looking at the therapeutic agency, attributes and potential of each of these facets in slightly more detail, highlighting where these key points intersect to serve the therapeutic goal, particularly with young children. I will start by looking at the spatial domain and then the material.

Therapeutic space and the 'spatiality' of puppetry

I have been influenced considerably by Paul Piris's ideas about the ontological ambiguity of the puppet (2015: 30-42). Piris outlines a useful conceptualisation of the self-other and subjective-objective pluralism as it manifests in puppetry performance, and he has in mind specifically those performances 'where visible manipulators interact with their puppets' as actors (Ibid., 30). Simply put, this ontological ambiguity exists because the relationship between self and other can only take place between two subjects. Since the puppet is an object, it receives its subject-ness through the puppeteer's manipulation and engagement with it, while, on the other hand, it does so through the spectators witnessing this interaction as a performance. This triangulation between puppet, puppeteer and spectator creates a shared space or mutual presence through which the actor's and puppet's identities are validated. In this setting, puppet, puppeteer and spectator achieve the symbolic synthesis of which I spoke earlier, through the extent to which the ontological ambiguities that characterise the relation between the three entities are resolved, essentially through their 'co-presence' (Ibid., 31). Or, in other words, the spatio-temporal manner in which they co-exist in the moment in the shared space within the theatre or performance space for the duration of the performance.

For Piris, the critical point in this process, which is simultaneously ethical and aesthetic, occurs through the 'puppetization' (Piris, 2015: 35) of the actor alongside the anthropomorphised or humanised puppet. This transformation occurs through the agency of the spectator's perception and imagination while watching the performance and, therefore, the extent to which this consciousness is in fact co-constitutive (and recursive) of the tripartite alliance within the performance space. Moreover, this process allows for the emancipation of the materiality of the puppet at the same time puppeteer and puppet co-exist in a newly constituted self-other intersubjectivity. In Piris's words:

> the puppeteer and the puppet appear co-present because spectators have the impression that they are witnessing two distinct subjects. This distinction results from the apparent presence of two bodies and two gazes on stage. (Ibid., 38)

When transposed to a dramatherapeutic setting, Piris's ideas have enormous validity and appeal – in particular, when clients engage directly with the puppet-making process and the creative imagination. Through the creative act and energy that the client brings to bear, he or she achieves at least two interrelated therapeutic outcomes. In the first instance, the client is able to recentre his or her internal locus of control and sense of self agency. In the second instance, as a result of the freedom to migrate between the materialisation and the embodiment that the puppet construction process affords, the client begins to establish a better understanding of the meaning and value of the world outside (i.e. the relational space) and of the ways in which the relationship with other manifest (i.e. the co-presence) and is negotiated in its exteriorised space. These therapeutic realisations (or insights) are of particular significance, for example, where any developmental changes or trauma the client has experienced may have dislodged one's capacity to feel in control, supported or safe.

Piris's thesis of ontological ambiguity and co-presence opens the door to an important theoretical avenue with regard to the pluralistic nature of the puppet and its therapeutic benefits that may have a significant impact on future dramatherapy research and practice. It is worth bearing it in mind before I move onto a discussion about the materiality of the puppet in the next sections of the chapter.

Earlier I referenced English scholar and object-oriented philosopher Timothy Morton's (2011, 2013) notion of 'interobjectivity'. In distinguishing between intersubjectivity and interobjectivity, Morton asserts that

> the phenomenon we call intersubjectivity is just a local, anthropocentric instance of a much more widespread phenomenon, namely interobjectivity … I [don't] mean something prior to or underneath or behind intersubjectivity. Think of intersubjectivity as a particular instance of interobjectivity with which humans are familiar. In other words, 'intersubjectivity' is really human interobjectivity with lines drawn around it to exclude nonhumans … We will find that all entities whatsoever are interconnected in an interobjective system. (2013, p. 69)

Morton makes the important point that interobjectivity encompasses all objects, including the 'non-sentient' and hence 'it explains phenomena such as social personhood', significant because 'it accounts for how change can occur, when sensual objects become entangled with one another' (2011).

Matt Smith, Applied Theatre practitioner from the University of Portsmouth's School of Art, Design and Performance, endorses this view:

> The main issue is that for too long we have ignored the objects in our practices and believed we were more significant. Adjusting this … makes better practice and a … fuller consideration of all the elements and networks. I am generally very interested in the ethics of objects and aspects of this … As a non-therapist I do not make claims about the benefits of

puppets in this way. Puppets are not tools but are co-collaborators in the space. They are wonderful bridging facilitators … in my practice I often say let the objects do the work.[2]

Once again, I believe that there is a rich seam of theoretical ideas being articulated by this school of thought that can significantly benefit dramatherapists working with young children and puppetry (and objects generally). By exploring this field practitioners will stretch their aesthetic, imaginative and psychodynamic vocabularies and interdisciplinary thinking in innovative and ground-breaking ways that may well contribute substantially to propagating new, emancipatory practice regimes. For instance, a strong case could be made for 'adjusting' some of the classic, over-determined psychoanalytic paradigms that still seem to hold so much sway. However, this may be the conversation for another occasion.

What does it/puppetry 'matter'

When I first began working with puppets therapeutically with young people, I would often bring a range of puppet samples that I had made to the sessions as a point of reference and stimulation for my clients. I would also bring a vast amount of materials, including huge assortments and quantities of paper, fabric and wool, glues, paints and paintbrushes, coloured pencils, string and adhesive tape. Typically, these were the materials I had used to make the puppets I had brought to the sessions. However, I quickly learnt to curb my exuberance and changed strategies as I had misgauged the age appropriateness of some of these items – for example, with the logistical impracticalities posed by using wet materials. More importantly, however, I had not factored into my planning that the children tended to see my puppet samples as the standard they had to aspire to and often this unspoken assumption on their part led to frustration when they felt they had fallen short in making their own puppets.

I have subsequently adopted a very different approach. I no longer take puppets samples into puppet-making sessions and, increasingly, I tend to use fewer and fewer materials. Those that I do use now tend to be of a very basic nature – for example, brown paper, cardboard and cardboard boxes, plastic bottles and some adhesive materials such as masking or gaffer tape – and frequently they tend to be recycled items.

The main therapeutic reason for adopting this strategy is based on the premise that the majority of clients in therapy are in need of support as a result of being alienated by and large from inner as well as outside resources to which they would possibly have access under different, less traumatic or disrupted circumstances. Therefore, working with a limited range of materials mimics this condition and approximates a tabula rasa situation, creating an opportunity to engage with the creative imagination in an unrestricted and regenerative manner that allows for the potential of any given piece of material to be made manifest.

However, there is an extremely important and more complex contextual consideration that underpins this clinical premise, my critical thinking and my research and practice approaches. It informs both the materials and the material techniques employed, as well as the material agencies and technologies at work when I engage in puppet-making sessions with my young clients. Moreover, it is strongly influenced by my anthropological and artistic interests as a social scientist and creative artist, as I suggested earlier when discussing my sources of inspiration from prehistoric rock art. Two influences are especially pertinent in this context: theatre historian, John Bell's (2008) insightful account of the evolving materiality of puppetry, mask and object theatre and its influence in the United States over the past 150 years; and anthropologist Norma Wolff's (2000) compelling study of the uses of human images in Yoruba medicine.

Bell (2008) reminds us that the wood, leather and bone from which traditional puppets and masks had been made over thousands of years were 'characterized by their connection to once-living materials' (Ibid., 219-220), to the spirits of the animals and the trees from which they derived. And through the performance becomes 'a kind of reinstallation of soul into once living matter' and accounts for 'part of its uncanny appeal' (Ibid.)

The emergence of new materials and technologies, such as plastic, glass, rubber, electricity and television, in the late nineteenth and twentieth centuries, was quickly assimilated into puppet and object theatre, resulting in their new hybrid forms and new performance spaces as exemplified so effectively and successfully in the United States through the use of rubber foam and the almost ubiquitous TV presence of Jim Henson's Muppets (Ibid., 221–224).

By contrast, Peter Schumann's Bread and Puppet Theater remained by choice, 'a "poor" theatre' relying on 'cheap building materials … cast-off lumber and other detritus' (Bell, 2008, p. 225). In this way, the company was able to maintain its freedom and autonomy to respond to the 'most important questions of the moment' and offer puppet performances 'with a decidedly political bent' (Ibid.).

There are three fundamental elements that Bell is underlining in his argument. Firstly, the 'payoff of live performance is not how many people are reached, but how profoundly they are reached' (Bell, 2008, p. 226, my emphasis). Secondly, the extent to which the 'simultaneous presence of humans and human-manipulated objects … create[s] an otherwise impossible artistic communion' that conveys 'a strength of communicative power that human beings alone cannot match' (Ibid., 226, 230). Thirdly, the combination of these points will enhance our ability to 'understand the powers of such materials in performance, in the context of … global cultures … [and] will be helpful to us for the rest of the century' (Ibid., 230).

Bell's claim that the recycling of materials through the performing object is a form of reconstituting and reinstating the 'soul into once living matter' at the same time that it preserves and perpetuates the same kinds of 'uncanny appeal' (Ibid., 220) and 'uncanny communicative powers' (2008,p. 230) over time and across cultures speaks strongly to the case I am making for the use of puppetry and puppet-making in dramatherapy settings.

Meanwhile, Norma Wolff's (2000) study on the use of human figures in Yoruba medicine anticipates a number of the themes Bell presents. Its specific alignment within the symbolic healing traditions (Moerman, 1979; Dow, 1986) and belief systems of many indigenous communities also provides another useful analogy for the aesthetic and therapeutic synthesis of the material and performative dimension of using the puppet dramatherapeutically. This is especially the case as far as we are concerned with the integration of the puppet-as-object and puppet-as-character tropes discussed previously.

Indigenous healers among the Yoruba of southwestern Nigeria, Wolff tells us,

> regularly utilize small carved and molded three-dimensional human figures in their medicines … [which] … are used by individuals in purposeful acts of magical mimesis to manipulate the social world.
>
> *(Wolff, 2000: 205)*

However, the figures themselves are not merely imitations, 'they are transformers that embody and channel the powers of the natural materials from which they are fashioned,' and their creation 'is an act of embodiment with the intention of concentrating powers of nature for social goals … [and] … to call forth and channel supernatural forces for the benefit of their owners' (Ibid., 207).

The figures are carved from wood or bone or moulded from clay, and since 'all of the natural world is a source of power … [they] … incorporate plant and animal parts and other natural objects, as well as artifacts, in varying combinations to draw upon the unique powers of each' (Ibid., 207). They are used 'to diagnose, cure, protect from, and, in some cases, cause illness and misfortune' (Ibid., 205). Their power lies in the instrumental role these objects play 'in channeling intangible supernatural forces for the benefit of individuals or the community' (Ibid., 207).

While the artists treat the themes of 'fecundity, productivity, youth, health, wealth, and power in single and group sculptures that portray everyday and important ritual activities' (Ibid., 208), the choice of materials used will depend on the practitioner's knowledge of 'the variegated personalities of the ingredients … [and on] … the goal to be achieved' (Ibid., 220). In addition, 'the medicine figures personalize and concretize specific latent powers of nature's forces as manifested in minerals, plants, animals, and spirit beings, so that the intangible takes human form' (Ibid., 220) and 'there is an interpenetration that bridges the natural, supernatural, and the social worlds' (Ibid., 222). Ultimately, the medicine figure 'reflects Yoruba beliefs about humans and their place in the larger universe' (Ibid., 221).

In many ways, the therapeutic intention through the metaphorical engagement with puppetry and puppet-making within dramatherapy practice, as with the Yoruba medicine figures, also attempts to reassert our sense of belonging and to reconnect us to the deeper truths and realities of our relational experience with others. However, it is important to underline the fact that Yoruba medicine is part of a complex belief system steeped in animism and that the medicine figures, no matter how suggestive, can only serve as an analogy for our purposes. Wolff, for example, reminds us that Yoruba medicine distinguishes between 'magic' and 'sorcery', that is, between benevolent and malevolent forces, respectively – both of which are fundamental elements of that belief system. It is difficult to conceive of a similar highly determined, rigid and ritualistically bonded moral and spiritual causality at work within dramatherapy settings outside of the metaphorical and aesthetic dimensions.

Of course, another important difference to point out is the fact that within the arts-based premises that underpin dramatherapy practice, the client–therapist alliance is much more symmetrical than in the Yoruba system. In particular, the client is actively invested and is probably at greater liberty to exercise his or her volition in the healing transaction, at the same time that it is the engaging through his or her creative imagination and creative expression that is central to the therapeutic process.

The use of puppets in therapeutic settings with young children is yet another, albeit highly specific and uniquely effective way for clients to engage with the creative imagination and creative expression to access and harness this polyvocality and agency in order to instil hope and, ultimately, to facilitate regeneration, change and healing.

Conclusion

In this chapter, I have attempted to explore aspects of the animating intelligence one brings to the therapeutic space through the creative production of the puppet-object when working dramatherapeutically with young people. I have probed the idea that the creative imagination and, through it, creative expression are among the most important resources we have for healing and, ultimately, that engaging clients in the puppet-making process offer a unique, albeit, neglected or under-used resource by most therapists including dramatherapists.

In my analysis, I theorised the puppet in terms of the artefact as a character and as an object, drawing on Piris's (2015) notion of the ontological ambiguity of the puppet and actor as a subjective and objective co-presence. Moreover, drawing on my inspiration from prehistoric rock art, as well as Bell's (2008) and Wolff's (2000) respective critiques of the materiality of the object as a performative and life-affirming symbol across diverse socio-cultural boundaries, I examined the inter-subjective and interobjective dynamic of the puppet in terms of some of its spatial and material dimensions and made a case for the correlations between our experience as human and spiritual beings and the extent to which the puppet can represent a symbolic link between these classifications.

I argued that through these dimensions, we can achieve a comprehensive synthesis of the spatial and material and, by extension, of the relationality between self and other, between internal and external loci of control – an integrational process that constitutes one of the most fundamental and important objectives of the therapeutic transaction.

Finally, I made an appeal to the dramatherapy professions in particular to fore-ground a more arts-based practice approach whereby it is the art form and the art practice itself that is the therapeutic catalyst and evidence rather than aspiring or conforming to over-determined empirically grounded medical explanatory models. I am convinced that by doing so, we will continue developing new and creative ways of addressing and staying ahead of the emergent and increasingly complex mental health challenges that face so many young people in the world today.

Acknowledgements

I would like to thank the following group of practitioners, puppeteers and other professionals active in the field of puppetry for their very generous support in helping to shape my ideas for this chapter: Cariad Astles, Chris Hill, Theodoris Kostadakis, Marilena Muratori, Chris Pirie, Claire Quigley, Matt Smith and Asa Viklund. All of these remarkable individuals are highly respected fellow professionals and peers in their respective fields in the UK and abroad, and I have had the pleasure and good fortune of having worked with all of them in some capacity – whether in training, teaching, performing or research.

Notes

1 The government information board at the iconic site declares that: 'Prehistoric peoples, probably from the Archaic, Basketmaker, Fremont and Pueblo cultures, etched on the rock from B.C. time to A.D. 1300. In historic times, Ute and Navajo people, as well as European Americans made their contributions. In interpreting the figures on the rock, scholars are undecided as to their meaning or have yet to decipher them. In Navajo, the rock is called "Tse' Hane" (rock that tells a story). Unfortunately, we do not know if the figures represent storytelling, doodling, hunting magic, clan symbols, ancient graffiti or something else. Without a true understanding of the petroglyphs, much is left for individual interpretation' (Reeve: n.d.).
2 Personal communication, 3rd October 2019.

References

Bell, J. (2008) *American puppet modernism: Essays on the material world of performance.* New York: Palgrave MacMillan.

Blumenthal, E. (2005) *Puppetry: A world history.* New York: Harry N. Abrams, Inc.

Dow, J. (1986) 'Universal aspects of symbolic healing: A theoretical synthesis', *American Anthropologist,* 88, pp. 56–69.

Jung, C.G. (1940) *The integration of the personality.* London: Kegan Paul, Trench, Trubner & Co.

Jurkowski, H. (2000) 'Among deities, priests and shamans (puppets within rituals)' in Fisher, J. (ed.) *The puppetry yearbook* (Vol. 4). Lewiston: The Edwin Mellen Press.

Moerman, D. (1979) Anthropology of symbolic healing. *Current Anthropology,* 20(1), pp. 59–80.

Morton, T. (2011) 'Ecology without nature' [Online]. Available at: http://ecologywithoutnature.blogspot.com/2011/03/interobjectivity.html [Accessed: 22 October 2019].

Morton, T. (2013) *Hyperobjects: Philosophy and ecology after the end of the world.* Minneapolis: University of Minnesota Press.

Piris, P. (2015) 'The co-presence and ontological ambiguity of the puppet' in Posner, D.N.,

Orenstein, C., and Bell, J. (eds.) *The Routledge companion to puppetry and material performance*. London: Routledge.

Reeve, P. (n.d.) 'Newspaper rock', *Utah Historical Markers* [Online]. Available at: https://utahhistoricalmarkers.org/c/sj/newspaper-rock/ [Accessed: 15 April 2020].

Stolfi, D. (2008) Dwelling between thresholds, *The puppet as intercessor: The use of puppetry as a dramatherapy medium with adult male offenders in a Category C prison setting*. Masters Dissertation. University of Plymouth.

Stolfi, D. (2011) 'Crossing thresholds: Therapeutic uses of puppetry as a dramatherapy medium with adult populations' in Scoble, S. (ed.) *The space in between*. Plymouth: University of Plymouth Press.

Wolff, N. (2000) 'The use of human images in yoruba medicines', *Ethnology*, 39(3), pp. 205–223.

4

DANCE MOVEMENT THERAPY WITH CHILDREN AND ADOLESCENTS

Rosemarie Samaritter

1 Introduction

Dance Movement Therapy (DMT) is a therapeutic method that aims to contribute to mental health, resilience and recovery from adversities through the use of dance, movement and body-oriented interventions. In DMT, therapeutic change is thought of in terms of changes in personal movement patterns and changes in movement actions shared between participants or between a participant and the therapist. All interventions employed by a dance/movement therapist are derived from dance-activities as are found in dance as socio-cultural practice. There is no culture without dance and often the younger generations develop and contribute with new modes of dance and movement to societal change. This phenomenon in modern times has been reflected in many dance films that introduced a new dance style and with it, often-times a new way of being or social identity. Dance therefore seems to be close to a younger population and may be specifically suitable to serve as a modality in the therapy for young people with psycho-social problems to express themselves and connect to others through the unique, yet universal language of movement.

Since the beginnings of DMT in the early 1940s, a broad diversity of methods has been developed for the mental health field and other, related fields. Among them are some approaches that specifically aim at supporting children and ado-lescents who are (at risk of) developing psycho-social pathologies.

This chapter offers a perspective to DMT in child and adolescent psychotherapeutic settings (CAPT) that has been informed by the DMT literature and by the author's more than 30 years clinical experience in outpatient CAPT. The first paragraph ad-dresses some overarching theoretical concepts and is followed by paragraphs providing insight in DMT theory and methods for CAPT. The chapter offers some examples from clinical practice with selected DMT applications for specific populations. Where applicable, the chapter also offers references to relevant research.

2 Therapy with children and adolescents

Therapy for children and adolescents always happens within developmental pathways. Throughout the development from new-born to adolescent, specific themes and issues occur, which, once mastered, contribute to building capacities in self-organisation and self-other-relatedness. The pathway from a new-born's dependency to the adolescents' autonomy is not just a linear continuity, but shows to be a close concert of inborn capacities, maturation, the richness of experiences and the systemic context in which they occur.

The development of meaningful moments and nourishing and supportive relations are core issues throughout human life. Research has shown that even before birth, the functioning of a child's organism and a child's development of interpersonal relating are deeply influenced by the rhythms and fluctuating tension in the shared maternal body (Provasi et al, 2014; Reissland and Kisilevsky, 2016). In the early developmental phases after birth, the body is the major means to communicate needs and to experience the caregiver(s). Newborns come into the world with an expertise on maternal/parental movement patterns as perceived through vital rhythms, circadian regulation and psychophysiological regulation during prenatal life. How this informedness will be processed throughout life will depend on the child's maturing capacities as well as on the environment's capacities to responsively attune to the child's needs.

In a complex interplay of congenital structures, maturation and experience, social emotional development is deeply bound to bodily/embodied processes. Through body-to-body interactions, the child learns about contact and relating to others and neuronal patterning will be formatted from these experiences (Meltzoff and Moore, 1998; Stern, 2002, 2010; Hobson and Hobson, 2008). The developmental tasks to be achieved vary from phase to phase and cover development of self-other differentiation, attachment and individuation, self-regulation and mentalisation (Fonagy et al., 2007). The child's development is in its very nature an intersubjective process, which emerges within and through the interaction with others. The relational experiences format patterns of functional connections in the social brain structures that contribute to the brain's capacity to read and predict intersubjective processes in future situations (De-Wit, Machilsen and Putzeys, 2010).

Disturbances throughout this development leading to specialist care or therapy can be grouped under three major clusters, which are related to

1. disturbances in the sensory/motor development (e.g. sensory processing/ sensory motor coordination/motor development),
2. disturbances in the development of sense of self (e.g. regulation/perception/ image/identity) and
3. disturbances in the development of self-other relationships (e.g. interpersonal engagement/interpersonal attunement/social cognition/intersubjectivity).

These three domains are closely intertwined and development throughout childhood tends to occur pervasively over the clusters. Therefore, any therapeutic approach for the treatment of children and adolescents preferably addresses these developmental domains in an integrative manner and will at times also involve caregivers/parents or peers for their role to the child's/adolescent's health and wellbeing (Barish, 2018). Dynamic movement experiences within the relational frame of therapist-child interactions or peer-to-peer-interactions as offered in DMT may be specifically suitable to serve the development of sensory-motor integration within a psycho-social context of self-other-relatedness. Combining an experiential methodology and systemic therapeutic perspective, DMT contributes to an experiential approach to the development of self, social competences and mentalisation (Di Paolo, De Jaegher and Rohde, 2010).

3 Dance movement therapy in child and adolescent psychotherapy – A theoretical model

DMT approaches with children and adolescents have a strong developmental and holistic orientation. DMT literature states that rather than focussing on the psychopathology, dance therapists will take the child's capacities as a point of departure for the therapy. Starting with the child's capacities to move, express and interact the dance therapist will engage the child in constructively affording (dance/movement) experiences that over time will lead towards the agreed treatment goals. DMT approaches in CAPT oftentimes have adapted psychotherapeutic frames of reference, with a preference of many therapists for a psycho-analytically informed therapy approach (e.g. Kestenberg, 1975; Eberhard-Kaechele, 2010), others focussing on attachment theories/patterns (e.g. Loman and Foley, 2003; Tortora, 2009) and intersubjectivity (Samaritter and Payne, 2013). Also, some DMT approaches in CAPT focus on a specific pathology, like trauma (e.g. Dunphy et al., 2014), autism (e.g. Kalish-Weiss, 2008; Devereaux, 2012; Koch et al., 2014; Samaritter, 2017), ADHD (e.g. Grönlund et al., 2005; Levin, 2016) or socio-emotional problems in medical conditions (e.g. Cohen and Walco, 1999; Tortora, 2019). Recent developments in DMT, do not only consider psychologically informed frames of reference for the construction of a DMT methodology for CAPT, but also seek to make more explicit use of specific working mechanisms that stem from dance as an art form and a form of social engagement (Koch, 2017). In order to apply these components to CAPT settings, the following paragraph will briefly summarise some of the core aspects of such a dance-informed approach.

3.1 Dance-informed core themes in CAPT

All dance forms can be understood as socio-cultural practices, which, despite their diversity of occurrences, show some generic characteristics. All dance practices are bound to the *embodied presence* of the dancers. For CAPT, body and movement serve as the source and means of sensations, feelings, experiences, actions and interactions but also integrate body organisation and coordination in the therapeutic context. While dancing, the body's *(neuro-)physiological regulatory mechanisms* are engaged in basic vital regulation, such as breathing rhythms and heart rate and rhythms of action and release. These aspects also play a major role in DMT; developing the body's animation and vitality are important themes in, for example, mood disorders, whereas neuro-physiological regulation plays a major role in treatment of anxiety disorders of posttraumatic disorders. Maybe the most recognised characteristic of dance is that it offers the opportunity to articulate experiential content through *symbolising movement and dance expression*, which may be developed into narrative structures like in a big ballet or in many primitive dances but also forms found in children's dance play. This aspect is helpful to support children towards creative expression and symbolisation of inner worlds. As in all dance forms, the *non-verbal interaction* between child and therapist in DMT takes place through movement qualities in space (e.g. proximity or distance), timing (e.g. synchronisation) and weight (e.g. engaging in each other's movement patterns). In DMT with children and adolescents, it is particularly important that all dance practices are embedded in a cultural context and that by adopting a specific way of dancing, participants synchronise and attune to this cultural context. Using elements in DMT from youth dance cultures, such as street dance or dance battles, anchors children and adolescents with developmental or psychological challenges naturally in their peer-group.

While dancing, movers are engaged in all these characteristics simultaneously. The synergy of embodiment, physiological regulation, expressed emotion, non-verbal interaction and cultural embeddedness in a single moment contributes to the *aesthetic quality* of the dance experience (Samaritter, 2018). For the therapeutic context in the work with children and adolescents, these characteristics may serve as guiding principles to compose activities that fit the child's personal needs and strengths whilst addressing the goals set for the therapeutic interventions.

The following vignette[1] shows the interwoven appearance of DMT components in a case of a 13-year-old girl with autism, for whom the treatment was meant to develop her communicative capacities and self-other-relatedness. The first phase of the DMT was characterised by movement material with patterns of strong spatial closure (e.g. making a personal spot, excluding the therapist from this spot -> finding individual body actions/embodiment), spatial orientation (e.g. moving through space without noticing/addressing the therapist's actions), connecting with the space around herself and an unfolding sensory-motor organisation. The vignette below is taken from a session that indicated a change in a girl who started to actively orient towards the other (i.e. therapist) and engage in instrumental interaction first with a prop, later also shifted to interactions through the prop with the therapist. (Box 4.1).

BOX 4.1   IN THIS VIGNETTE, THE DMT CORE THEMES ARE INDICATED AS FOLLOWS: EMBODIMENT (EB), PHYSIO-LOGICAL REGULATION (PR), EXPRESSED EMOTIONS (EE), NON-VERBAL INTERACTION (NI) AND CULTURAL SYNCH-RONISATION (CS). NOTICE THAT ALL ASPECTS ARE AT WORK SIMULTANEOUSLY DURING DANCE ACTIVITIES; ONLY THE CORE THEME THAT IS ON THE FOREGROUND OF INTERACTION AND INTERVENTION IS INDICATED IN BRACKETS

The girl has chosen a fan to work with. Initially she goes with the instrumental aspects of the prop, opening and closing it (EB), fanning herself some air into the face (PR), working individually with the material in a spatial closure, constituting kinesphere (EB). After a while, she also starts to address the therapist in a similar use of the material and interacts on this instrumental level (fanning, interplay opening closing) and doing so, interacting from her personal space towards the therapist (NI). The therapist on her part answers these instrumental actions, whilst in addition taking a very vertical movement attitude (EB), through which she is referring to the body attitude that is seen in dances that use a fan such as Spanish flamenco or dances from the Baroque era (CS). Also, she covers her face every now and then with the fan (NI). The girl starts to pick up responsively the vertical body attitude (EB), integrating the fan now into full body movement. In this context, the fan is no longer an instrumental attribute but serves as prolongation of arm movements and with that she accentuates and increases personal space (EB). Initially mimicking the therapists dance attitude (NI), she later shifts into more sudden and direct movement qualities, that bring a fighting character to the dance (EE). And indeed, from this shift in movement quality, she starts to build an aesthetic illusive dance in which she fights the therapist and 'chasses' her across the room (EE/NI/CS). The therapist, in turn, without losing her strength answers within the aesthetic illusion with soft, mouldable movement qualities, which allow for the participant to fully explore the options of a powerful attitude towards the adult (NI/EB/CS/EE). When the dancers move unto a wall (external stimulus), the girl seems to change into a different movement engagement and shift of movement quality accordingly. The dance ends with a release of the fighting quality into a more playful interaction (PR/NI/EE).

3.2 Dance-informed working procedures

The described components may occur in various dance-related procedures. Imagine how dancers *invite* their co-dancers onto the dance floor or the audience to the dance performance and seek to *engage* them in the dance activity. Similarly, the therapist will look for suitable procedures to invite the child into the dance space and engage it in the movement experience. Dancers *explore* the movement elements/ patterns involved in the dance and *play* with variations or ways of practicing. These dance procedures of exploration and play are close to the child's approach of the world and as such they are useful in a therapeutic context. Experiential structures modulate through childhood and adolescence according to the child's developmental phase. Being well at home with a broad variety of dance forms allows the therapist to playfully create a suitable dance world for the individual child. In this process, therapist and child interact within and through movement. While dancing, they are directly and kinaesthetically informed by their own movements and those of their movement partners. This way, every dance situation is a co-creation on the spot. Like all dancers, they know instantly through their kinaesthetic senses about one another and co-create an intersubjective space, which is maintained through the shared dance activities and movement materials. To create a dance form or choreography, dancers not only need playfulness and creativity to explore suitable movement material but also need to select movements, repeat them and adjust, put them together, compose meaningful structures. These activities are paralleled in the therapeutic setting with finding new perspectives and alternative action patterns, addressing other emotional worlds than conflict and change of harmful patterns. In this process, *changes* are produced through the dancer's constant kinaesthetic awareness and responsive movement adjustments to the emerging movement material. These processes are driven by reflecting on the meaningfulness of specific movement material for a chosen theme, and decision making on the suitability of the movement material for a specific sequence, occasion or narrative. Choreographing the found material into structures that are replicable finally leads to performance, such as in shared spontaneous choreographies (instant composing) or in improvisational pieces or set pieces which require performativity, embodied presence, executive functioning in performing the chosen movement material and memorising the choreography. During a performance, the observers are addressed as witness of the dance, in case of therapy, the empathetic observation of group members and therapist. These structures basically cover embodied engagement and address creativity and aesthetic involvement, which offer a possibility to enter a realm that allows for shaping a situation to the needs as well as the capacities of the child and allow for them to build whatever might be needed to bring about support or change for the better. The following vignette shows the dynamic use of dance-informed procedures in the starting phase of a dance therapy with an eight-year-old boy who has been diagnosed with multiple developmental disorders, resulting in non-regulated, very impulsive behaviours, which were not accessible to external regulation by a parent or other care giver (Box 4.2).

BOX 4.2   IN THIS VIGNETTE, SOME PROCEDURAL ASPECTS ARE INDICATED IN ITALICS IN BRACKETS

An eight-year-old boy comes into the relatively large therapy room, that is provided by the school for children with special needs he is attending. He immediately starts to move around impulsively (*experiment/play*). He is not able to contain or regulate his movements and seems to 'fall apart'. He doesn't address or interact with the therapist. Any attempts on the side of the therapist (*invite*) to help him regulate his movement result in defensive avoidance on the side of the child (*interact*). The therapist discusses with the parents the option to move to another, smaller and less furnished therapy space outside the school environment to which they agree. In the smaller room, the boy responds with calmer movement engagement (*play*), although still heavily dysregulated at times, he starts walking the space (without paying attention to the therapist) (*replicate*). Eventually, he starts citing dialogues from a computer game he knows very well and plays frequently (*replicate*). The therapist follows in his pathways and over time is addressed by the boy as if she would be another figure in the play (*interact/play/change*). From this imitative aesthetic illusion, the two of them keep walking (*replicate*), with the therapist very responsive to the contents of the spoken words, but also very attentive for moments that allow for little changes to be applied in the movement qualities (*change*), like giving more weight into a movement and from there bouncing into a jump (after which the boy picks up the aesthetic mimicking again), or they occur as changes in the constellation between child and therapist, for example, holding hands while walking, which allows for slight changes in the shared timing by slowing down or accelerating tempo (*replicate/change/improvise*). Both examples show options of putting a real-time element to the aesthetic reproduction of the game scenery. In the following sessions, real-time interaction increases and eventually dominates the sessions (*improvisation/play*), although the mimicking re-occurs every now and then it also seems that within that game, the interactions not only replicate what is happening in the computer game, but also get a new contents, that stems from the movement interaction between child and therapist (*improvisation/play*), within the continuation of the given phantasy characters. In the real interaction between child and therapist, the movement qualities develop into playful encounters, in which moving together in shared movement qualities develops towards turn taking and finally also towards performativity in that the boy shows little movement sequences or little movement scenes/narratives to the therapist (*compose/present*), who has to act a responsive audience, or is invited, in turn, to show a little movement sequence to the boy. It seems that initially the smaller movement space and then the aesthetic frame of the computer game and later the performances act like a holding environment for this boy to start to engage in the real encounter with the therapist and explore other than the well-known behaviour patterns. While he wasn't able to contain himself in the first environment, he is able to develop towards self-containment and self-regulation through the aesthetic structure of entering the 'game space' and within that develop towards real-time interaction with the therapist.

On the background of the described general characteristics of DMT as describe through core themes and procedures, the following paragraphs will focus on some specific aspects of DMT in the treatment of children and adolescents.

4 DMT with the developing child: The role of movement observation

Therapists emphasise that DMT should always carefully join the child's movement capacities and movement patterns. With ongoing movement analysis, the therapist monitors the child's movement behaviours. Dance/movement therapists usually use observational methods that are based on Laban Movement Analysis (LMA) (Laban, 1980). Specifically, for the analysis of movement behaviours of young children and their care givers, Judith Kestenberg developed in the early 1970s the Kestenberg Movement Profile (KMP) (Kestenberg-Amighi et al., 1999). The KMP specifically considers that movement patterns are subject to development and occur in successive phases. The strength of LMA and KMP is that they both inventory the movement patterns as they occur at a specific moment in time and therefore are highly sensitive to the child's specific developmental level. The dance/movement therapist summarises the observed movement patterns in a movement profile.

The therapist will shape interventions on the background of the movement profile as a picture of the whole scope of the child's movement capacities, re-occurring or frozen movement patterns. Sensory-motor organisation and engagement are involved throughout all movement activities.

All movement can serve as a starting point and will be met by the therapist responsively with an experiential deepening or modulation of the movement patterns by changing, for example, just one movement aspect/element, like changing the rhythm of a movement pattern (slowing down or speeding up), or changing the direction of movement. Through the continuous movement analysis, the therapist is able to also capture and support spontaneous (movement) initiatives of the child or spontaneous new (movement) behaviours. The therapist will invite the child into movement experiences that are within or close to the child's mastery of movement capacities. To support therapeutic change and provoke new behaviours, the dance/movement therapist may invite the child into slightly challenging movement situations but will do so with the child's developmental potential taken into account.

Movement observation allows for a flexible response by the therapist, regardless any developmental delays, psychological or psychiatric problems in the child. This way, DMT is also very suitable for children with sensory-/psycho-motor delays or atypical developmental patterns, which often co-occur with socio-emotional issues. Dance therapy can thus address the child in a non-pathologising way and offer a supporting, nurturing context for the child to shift into a constructive, healthy development. However, it is important to carefully monitor the child's movement profile, including functional, sensory-motor development.

Also, the child's movement material serves as a starting point for improvisations around creative explorations, expressive variations and symbolisation that the child brings to the therapy situation. Developing and choreographing personal movement sequences allow for the therapist to address the experiential aspect of kinetic material, in terms of emotional content, movement narratives or intersubjective engagement. Within this holistic context of moving and being moved, playing with own impulses and those coming from the environment, the child's sensory-motor organisation is playfully orientated towards the movement situation, which is tailored by the therapist such as to invite change and broaden and develop the child's expressive, emotional and intersubjective capacities over time. The therapist will comprehensively integrate the child's initiatives in dance-informed procedures and integrate them in the aesthetic context of aforementioned core themes.

The individual development may also be integrated in systemic or group approaches (Bender, 2014; Wengrower, 2015) to offer the possibility for the child to integrate interpersonal experiences with care givers or peers.

In the literature on DMT in CAPT, the observation of interpersonal movement behaviours has been given some attention. Some authors also offer specific observational tools/methods for the observation of a single child within the context of a group or family therapy (Dulicai, 2010).

5 The central role of the non-verbal therapeutic relationship in dance movement therapy

In all DMT methods for children or adolescents, the central role of the non-verbal therapeutic relation has been emphasised by the authors. The relation between therapist and child develops in dance movement therapy in non-verbal, shared movement experiences that are monitored by the therapist with ongoing movement observation from which he or she will take cues for further interventions. Active interpersonal attunement, initially introduced one-sidedly by the therapist, offers the opportunity to develop and support the child's capacities to relate to others. While very much on the foreground in parent–child interactions throughout childhood and adolescence, attunement processes underlie all human interaction until death. In interplay with the developmental changes, nonverbal attunement patterns are shifting contingently over the life span. Although they shift more to the background in adulthood, they inform intersubjective interactions on the mutual relatedness in essential ways. In the early dyadic interaction between caregivers and their children and in cases of neurodegenerative disorders, such as dementia, they often form the only option for intersubjective engagement (Beebe and Lachmann, 2003).

The child's dyadic interaction may be severely influenced/disturbed in cases of atypical development of the child. Parenting strategies may not answer the child's specific needs, for example, in cases of attention or hypersensitivity disorders and autism. The child's a-typical behaviours also may have an impact on the attunement behaviours of their interaction partners. Hobson and Hobson (2008) showed that reduced levels of non-verbal interaction coming from the child/adolescent with ASD led to reduced non-verbal engagement in the neuro-typical interaction partner, hence the opportunities to engage mutually seemed to be significantly reduced in neuro-typical and neurodivergent mixed dyadic interactions.

Psychopathology in a parent or a problematic family situation can also have an impact on the subtle intersubjective attunement processes in the interactions between children and caregivers. The early dyad seems to be very sensitive to heightened stress levels in the care giver (Loughlin, 2009). Papousek and Papousek (1997) showed already in the 1990s that the infant in interaction with a depressed mother tends to disengage from the interaction, for example, by looking away, and on a very basic bodily level, tends to disorganise in the organisation of the body after not being met with full attuned engagement (visible in loss of navel radiated actions).

It should be considered that children who have experienced violence or abuse may respond in the therapy situation with strong withdrawal or behavioural dysregulation. In these cases, a highly attuned therapist responsiveness can be overwhelming for the child's affected attunement system/capacities. Here, dance therapists can make a specific contribution through their highly tailored intervention to the child's non-verbal interactions. Making use of movement analysis, the therapist will look for a shared point of departure within the movement interaction that suits the child's capacities to relate. The KMP is suitable to focus on subtle interaction through shifting flows of body tension and shape. Also, DMT as re-nurturing and re-socialising intervention needs to integrate the systemic embeddedness of a child and will therefore seek the collaboration with parents or caregivers with the intention to improve intersubjective attunement in the daily life context.

5.1 Relational modes

In the literature, dance therapists describe how they carefully build the working relation with the participants through non-verbal attunement and relational movement structures. The dance therapist will tailor the non-verbal attunement closely to child's needs to connect or distance and intentions to interact within the shared movement situation. Close reading of the DMT literature in CAPT shows some commonalities in how dance therapists intervene in the therapeutic relation. The author has proposed the use of *relational modes* to capture the relational interventions applied in DMT. The following paragraph describes some of these modes more in detail.

A very popular relational mode is *joint movement*, in which the therapist joins into the movement repertoire of the child without expecting the child to respond to the non-verbal attunement or relational structure. In this mode, the therapist takes the actions of the child as a contribution to the shared movement situation, whether or not the child shows an interactional intention. The most common intervention in this mode is that of *mirroring* the movements of the child. Mirroring here is understood as responsively picking up on the child's movement patterns rather than imitating them strictly. The therapist will pick up the child's movement patterns and, in order to promote experiential engagement, will deepen their quality by, for example, enlarging the spatial characteristics, speeding up the tempo of the movement or giving more weight to a movement impulse. Some authors describe specific variations of mirroring interventions, related to the developmental phase of the child (e.g. Eberhard-Kaechele, 2010) or the phase of the therapy (e.g. Loman and Foley, 2003; Tortora, 2009). However, all the variations of mirroring share the one-sided intentional attunement of the therapist towards child. Another example of *joint movement* is the intervention of *shadowing*, during which the therapist follows the movements of the child responsively, keeping track with the child during spatial explorations, without necessarily picking up on the movement patterns as such. Where mirroring is oriented mainly to the movement qualities, shadowing is mainly oriented on the spatial relationship between child and therapist.

Another relational mode described by dance therapists in the CAPT is that of *leading/following*. All variations of this mode are organised similarly to structures of *follow the leader*, which are present in children's (dance) games of many cultures. In DMT, the therapist may pick up the movement of a child and show how she follows the child's guidance. This intervention is often applied in circle formations like, for example, in the Chace work. This relational mode offers a strong containment for children who do not have an idea on how to move or who dare not present their own movement material or explore space. On the other hand, shifts in leadership may invite the child to explore a new role, such as taking the responsibility of leading another person or regulating oneself to the movement guidance of a partner.

A third relational mode is the *empathetic observation*. Originally developed within the method of authentic movement (Adler, 2003), this mode allows for the therapist to stay out of direct movement interaction with the child and take the role of an observer or *witness*, who is empathetically involved and responsive to the child's movement material through *kinaesthetic listening* (Petitmengin-Peugeot, 1999). This mode is especially applied to offer the child the space to develop and explore personal themes or movement material, without having to take the therapist's (or group members') movement responses or personal explorations into account. This may apply in improvisational phases or situations where a child is building a personal movement world (e.g. creating a landscape for movement stories). Also, it may apply in therapies where the child is not used or able to engage in continuous non-verbal attunement and interaction, as could be the case, for example, in autism or social anxiety disorders. There, this mode can offer a space for individual movement experiences without loss of holding containment by the therapist.

Finally, the most intersubjective relational mode would be the *movement dialogue*, in which child and therapist move together in continuous interaction. In this relational mode, the movers are oriented towards and engaged in the shared movement situation. Whilst improvising from their personal movement material, they contribute to the shared movement patterns developing between them and are conscious agents in the process of co-creating the shared situation.

All relational modes have in common that they allow for working with and from the child's individual movement material, emotional material and interactional capacities. Throughout the dance therapy, the working relation will shift between the different modes according to the set goals and demands of the actual therapy situation.

The following vignette gives an impression on the change of relational modes during a DMT session with a 15-year-old boy with severe social anxiety disorder in comorbid dissociative disorder (Box 4.3).

Intersubjective dance and movement experiences between child and therapist are understood to contribute to a sense of self-other relatedness that is informed by sensory/motor experiences. Sensations coming from the body during movement activities are experienced as perception of oneself, for example, through the spatial experience of personal space, or personal boundaries of oneself and the movement partners in movement experiences with a prop. When changing the shared movement situation through their individual motor action, participants can experience a sense of agency within the shared activities.

5.2 Reflexivity

While moving, there may also be verbal exchange, commenting on the movement process as a whole or single moment. Verbalisation of movement behaviours may support the child's cognitive understanding of the doings. More reflective verbal interventions may support mentalisation on changes that occur of may support the child's identification with their individual contribution to the shared movement situation. The child's own verbal expressions on the other hand may promote enactive reflection and hermeneutically interpret movement processes in view of their meaningfulness for the child's self-image (in adolescents, identity) and mental representation of the lived experience. Through these reflexive activities, the therapy is taken towards integration of body perception, movement experience and life story (Habermas and Köber, 2015).

BOX 4.3 IN THIS VIGNETTE, SOME RELATIONAL MODES ARE INDICATED THROUGHOUT THE TEXT, WHILST DESCRIBING THE ACTION WITHIN THE CONTEXT OF CORE THEMES AND PROCEDURES

A 15-year-old boy is sitting with the therapist at the table in the movement space. After the introduction, the therapist asks where in space he would like to start. He tells her that he can see them standing there (a chair in between them). Asked for further explanation he tells her that he knows that he is standing there with her, but that he actually doesn't feel himself standing there, instead, he feels himself standing approximately one metre behind his actual position. This way he is not really present in the position that the therapist and others are addressing their actions to. He is, as it is, hidden for the interaction partner. This form of disembodiment, with a tendency to completely dissociate from embodiment, helps him to cope with his deep social anxiety. The DMT therapist shifts to some spatial distance and to the mode of empathetic witnessing with kinaesthetic listening. She invites the boy to explore the space in a way that feels comfortable for him. After a while she suggests him to create a spot that could serve as a home base, a spot that is only meant for him to access. Starting with some small, orienting movement impulses, he finally ends up in a spot in the periphery of the room, following the suggestion of the therapist to make a spatial closure by delineating the personal spot with a rope. From this, the therapist offers suggestions that are related to spatial compositions which allow for him to be present without being in direct interaction with the therapist, who stays contingently in the empathetic observation. Movement suggestions by the therapist are related to having a personal spot leading to the idea of a personal (uninhabited) island. Eventually, the boy is able to leave the spot with short distances, then returning and through this action small loops of structured time emerge. The therapist carefully starts to join into shadowing on the side of the client). Eventually, he engages in short encounters when their paths cross. With the crossing being an option rather than an obligation, the boy has a choice to regulate whether or not he will meet the therapist on one of his pathways (agency and regulation with regards to interaction). From the initial gestural greeting at crossings (gestural movement dialogue), they develop towards more (weight-) engagement and short improvisational loops around the theme 'meet and greet' (fully engaged movement dialogue). According to his self-report, the boy is able to stay within his real-body boundaries (embodiment) during these dance improvisations.

6 Conclusion

The discussed elements of DMT core themes, procedures and relational modes offer the possibility to tailor dance and movement structures that can specifically address the developmental problems that bring children and adolescents into CAPT.

The non-interpretive movement observation that the dance/movement therapist brings to the therapeutic context offer a distinctive diagnostic contribution to the treatment planning in CAPT.

The body-relatedness that is in the very nature of DMT offers multiple options to address and support sensory-/motor development within the embeddedness of creative and aesthetic experiences.

Moving with attention and awareness for signals coming from the body, the interoceptive and kinaesthetic information is processed as being self-related. Moving with a partner, the perception of being with the other in space and time, engaging intentionally in the shared movement activities, may heighten the awareness for relational movement markers, like orienting towards the partner, engaging in shared movement qualities or synchronising in movement rhythms and phrasing (Samaritter, 2017).

DMT offers a broad variety of treatment options for children and adolescents to live through new experiences. Repeated positive body and movement experiences cluster to patterns, that through repetition over time will form recognisable structures and will pattern into the child's neuro-/psychophysiological organisation. Due to their embodied quality, these experiences will easily transfer to situations other than the therapeutic context and will thus inform behaviours in daily life situations. Involving the systemic context through family therapy or group therapy is strongly recommended to support the participants socio-emotional and socio-cultural integration.

Note

1 All clinical vignettes in this chapter have been composed to illustrate a specific topic. They are based on the clinical experience of the author in child and adolescent psychiatric outpatient settings of a Dutch National Mental Health Institution. It is always difficult to capture a case in a brief vignette and to cover the developmental process throughout a therapy or the embeddedness of a DMT in other treatment or systemic aspects. The little vignettes throughout this text are meant to provide the reader with an experiential perspective to the contents. They are in no way meant to cover the complete treatment.

References

Adler, J. (2003) 'From autism to the discipline of authentic movement. 37th Annual Conference Keynote Address', *American Journal of Dance Therapy,* 25(1), pp. 5–16.

Barish, K. (2018) Cycles of understanding and hope: Toward an integrative model of therapeutic change in child psychotherapy⋆. *Journal of Infant, Child & Adolescent Psychotherapy,* 17(4), pp. 232–242. https://doi.org/10.1080/15289168.2018.1526022

Beebe, B., and Lachmann, F. (2003) The relational turn in psychoanalysis: A dyadic systems view from infant research. *Contemporary Psychoanalysis*, 39(3), pp. 379–409.

Bender, S. (2014) *Systemische Tanztherapie*. München: Ernst Reinhardt.

Cohen, S.O., and Walco, G.A. (1999) 'Dance/movement therapy for children and adolescents with cancer', *Cancer Practice*, 7(1), pp. 34–42.

Devereaux, C. (2012) 'Moving into relationships. Dance/Movement therapy with children with autism' in Gallo-Lopez, L., and Rubin, L. (eds.) *Play-based interventions for children and adolescents with autism spectrum disorders*. New York: Routledge.

De-Wit, L., Machilsen, B., and Putzeys, T. (2010) Predictive coding and the neural response to predictable stimuli. *Official Journal of the Society for Neuroscience*, 30(26), pp. 8702–8703. doi: 10.1523/JNEUROSCI.2248-10.2010

Di Paolo, E., De Jaegher, H., and Rohde, M. (2010) 'Horizons for the enactive mind: values, social interaction, and play' in Stewart, J, Gapenne, Ol., and Di Paolo, E. (eds.) *Enaction: Towards a new paradigm for cognitive science*. Cambridge: MIT Press, pp. 33–87.

Dulicai, D. (2010) 'Movement assessment of families: A system model' in Bender, S. (ed.) *Movement analysis of interaction/Bewegungsanalyse von Interaktionen*. Berlin: Logos.

Dunphy, K., Elton, M., and Jordan, A. (2014) 'Exploring dance/movement therapy in post-conflict Timor-Leste', *American Journal on Dance Therapy*, 36, pp. 189–208.

Eberhard-Kaechele, M. (2010) 'Spiegelungsvorgänge in der Tanztherapie/Körperpsychotherapie' in Bender, S. (ed.), *Bewegungsanalyse von Interaktion – Movement Analysis of Interaction*. Berlin:Logos, pp. 193–212.

Fonagy, P., Gergely, G., and Target, M. (2007) 'The parent–infant dyad and the construction of the subjective self', *Journal of Child Psychology and Psychiatry*, 48, pp. 288–328. 10.1111/j.1469-7610.2007.01727.x

Grönlund, E., Renck, B., and Weibull, J. (2005) 'Dance/movement therapy as an alternative treatment for young boys diagnosed as ADHD: A pilot study', *American Journal for Dance Therapy*. doi: 10.1007/s10465-005-9000-1

Habermas, T., Köber, C. (2015) 'Autobiographical reasoning is constitutive for narrative identity: The role of the life story for personal continuity' in Mclean, K.C., and Syed, M. (eds.) *The Oxford handbook of identity development*. Oxford: Oxford University Press, pp. 149–165.

Hobson, R.P., and Hobson, J.A. (2008) 'Dissociable aspects of imitation: a study in autism', *Journal of Experimental Child Psychology*, 101(3), pp. 170–185.

Kalish-Weiss, B.I. (2008) The case of Richard: Assessment and analytic treatment of a two-year-old twin with autistic-like states. *Journal of Infant, Child & Adolescent Psychotherapy*, 7(1), pp. 37–57. 10.1080/15289160701382303

Kestenberg, J. (1975) *Children and parents*. New York: Jason Aronson.

Kestenberg-Amighi, J., Loman, S., Lewis, P., and Sossin, K.M. (1999) *The meaning of movement: Developmental and clinical perspectives of the Kestenberg Movement Profile*. Amsterdam: Gordon & Breach.

Koch, S. (2017) 'Arts and health: Active factors and a theory framework of embodied aesthetics', *Arts Psychotherapy*, 54, pp. 85–91.

Koch, S.C., Mehl, L., Sobanski, E., Sieber, M., and Fuchs, T. (2014) 'Fixing the mirrors: A feasibility study of the effects of dance movement therapy on young adults with autism spectrum disorder', *Autism*, 19(3), pp. 338–350. 10.1177/1362361314522353

Laban, R. (1980) *The mastery of movement*. 4th edn, revised and enlarged by L. Ullmann. London: MacDonald and Evans. (First published as *The mastery of movement on the stage*, 1950).

Lagerlöf, I., and Djerf, M. (2009) 'Children's understanding of emotion in dance', *European Journal of Developmental Psychology*, 6(4), pp. 409–431. 10.1080/17405620701438475

Levin, K. (2016) 'Aesthetics of hyperactivity: A study of the role of expressive movement in ADHD and capoeira', *American Journal on Dance Therapy*, 38, pp. 41–62.

Loman, S., and Foley, L. (2003) 'Models for understanding the nonverbal process', *Arts Psychotherapy*, 23(4), pp. 341–350. 10.1016/0197-4556(96)00005-6

Loughlin, E. (2009) 'Intuitive mothering: Developing and evaluating a dance therapy model for mothers with postnatal depression and their vulnerable infants', *Dance Therapy Collections*, 3 ©DTAA.

Meltzoff, A.N., and Moore, M. (1998) 'Infant intersubjectivity: Broadening the dialogue to include imitation, identity and intention' in Bråten, S. (ed.) *Intersubjective communication and emotion in early ontogeny*. Cambridge Cambridge University Press, pp. 47–63.

Papousek, H., and Papousek, M. (1997) 'Fragile aspects of early social interaction' in Myrray, L., and Cooper, P.J. (eds) *Post-partum depression and child development*. New York: Guilford Press, pp. 35–53.

Petitmengin-Peugeot, C. (1999) 'The intuitive experience' in Varela, F., and Shear, J. (eds.) *View from within First person approaches to consciousness*. London: Imprint Academic, pp. 43–77.

Provasi, J., Anderson, D., and Barbu-Roth, M. (2014) 'Rhythm perception, production, and synchronization during the perinatal period', *Frontiers in Psychology*, 5, p. 1048. doi: 10.3389/fpsyg.2014.01048

Reissland, N., and Kisilevsky, B.S. (eds.) (2016) *Fetal development: Research on brain and behavior, environmental influences, and emerging technologies*. Cham, Switzerland: Springer. doi: 10.1007/978-3-319-22023-9_8

Samaritter, R. (2017) 'Shared movement: A dance-informed contribution to non-verbal interpersonal relating in autism spectrum disorders', in Payne, H. (ed.) *Essentials of dance movement psychotherapy: International perspectives on theory, research, and practice*. London: Routledge/Taylor & Francis Group, pp. 112–128.

Samaritter, R. (2018) 'The aesthetic turn in mental health: Reflections on an explorative study into practices in the arts therapies', *Behavioural Sciences*, 8, p. 41. doi: 10.3390/bs8040041.

Samaritter, R., and Payne, H. (2013) 'Kinaesthetic intersubjectivity: A dance informed contribution to self-other-relatedness and shared experience in non-verbal psychotherapy with an example from autism', *Arts Psychotherapy*, 40(1), pp. 143–150. doi: 10.1016/j.aip.2012.12.004

Stern, D.N. (2002) *The first relationship: Infant and mother*. Cambridge, MA: Harvard University Press.

Stern, D.N. (2010) *Forms of vitality. Exploring dynamic experience in psychology, the arts, psychotherapy and development*. Oxford: Oxford University Press.

Tortora, S. (2009) 'Dance/movement psychotherapy in early childhood treatment' in Chaiklin, S., and Wengrower, H. (eds.) *The art and science of dance/movement therapy*. London: Routledge.

Tortora, S. (2019) 'Children are born to dance! Pediatric medical dance/movement therapy: The view from integrative pediatric oncology', *Children*, 6(1), p. 14. doi: 10.3390/children6010014

Wengrower, H. (2015) 'Dance movement therapy groups for children with behavioral disorders' in Kourkoutas, E., and Hart, A. (eds.) *Innovative practice and interventions for children and adolescents with psychosocial difficulties and disabilities*. Cambridge/Newcastle Upon Tyne, UK: Cambridge Scholar Publications, pp. 390–414.

5

PARTICIPATORY ETHNOGRAPHY TO EXPLORE THE RELEVANCE OF CULTURAL ARTS PRACTICES TO THE PSYCHOSOCIAL WELLBEING OF ADOLESCENTS AFFECTED BY VIOLENCE IN TRINIDAD AND TOBAGO

Sarah Soo Hon

Introduction

The highest levels of homicide among children and adolescents have been recorded in the regions of Latin America and the Caribbean (UNICEF, 2014), with the impact of violence on adolescents observed to include, lethal and non-lethal injuries, long-term mental and emotional negative effects, decreased academic performance and heightened risks of engaging in violent behaviour (Office of the SRSG on Violence against Children, 2016). A Global School-based health survey conducted in Trinidad and Tobago among students, ages 13–15, also indicated that 33.6% of students were involved in one or more physical fights over the course of a year (World Health Organization, 2017).

While previous studies have examined the effects of violence on adolescents (Office of the SRSG on Violence against Children, 2016) and community risk factors leading to increased violence among youth (Williams and Van Dorn, 1999), there is limited research that involves participatory methods with youth on issues of violence in Trinidad and Tobago, particularly in the form of in-depth, qualitative research (Adams, Morris and Maguire, 2018). Additionally, research that identifies the potential benefits of arts and art therapy interventions with youth at risk and those affected by violence (Farnum and Schaffer, 1998; Freytes Frey and Cross, 2011; Office of Education and Culture/DHDEC, Executive Secretariat for Integral Development Organization of American States, 2011; Malchiodi, 2014), while extensive, do not accommodate for the historical, temporal, cultural or socio-political context of Trinidad and Tobago, and this presents challenges in their application. Hocoy (2002) points out, for example, that art therapy may utilise psychological constructs, which are not valid cross-culturally. Furthermore, assumptions about identity, family and community relationships, access to resources, as well as the significance and meaning of symbols in art therapy are predominantly Euro-American in origin and may undermine the relevance and effectiveness of art therapy interventions for individuals of differing backgrounds.

Socio-cultural context

Hall (1997) proposes that culture and cultural identity are concepts, which are constantly transforming representations and meanings. Understanding culture in Trinidad and Tobago requires not only reflection, and investigation into how people recognise or adopt shared concepts, but also how these concepts are experienced in ways that help people communicate and make sense of the world. As a post-colonial, independent and sovereign state, cultural identity in Trinidad and Tobago not only references a particular historical past, but also consists of current, transforming and increasingly fragmented identities, which are also partly reconstructed and reimagined from history, language, culture, fantasy and symbolism (Hall, 1996).

The islands of Trinidad and Tobago are former colonies of the British Empire. It gained independence in 1962, and was recognised as a Republic in 1976, after a lengthy history of colonisation as a plantation economy. Enslaved and indentured labour fuelled the agricultural industries of sugar and cocoa, shaped patterns of migration (Horne, 2003) and perpetuated the use violence as a means of power and control well into the post-independence period (Brereton, 2010).

Post-slavery and into the twentieth century, Trinidad and Tobago experienced rapid socio-economic development, which attracted rural-to-urban and intra-Caribbean migration to its capital city of Port of Spain. Social repercussions of this growth resulted in the development of unplanned settlements and poor living conditions, particularly in nearby areas such as Laventille. However, Laventille did not benefit from schemes implemented to improve infrastructure, and by the 1860s, it already established a reputation as a crime-stricken community with high levels of unemployment (Ryan et al., 1997). This community continues to struggle with many socio-economic ills, in the modern day, and has become the focus of this study as a community representative of one that is affected by everyday violence.

Bourdieu's concept of habitus argues that historical, societal and political conditions inform the habits and actions of people, through a relational understanding of the struggle for power within the structure of social settings (Swartz, 1997). Habitus implicitly guides many systems of practice such as social class, marriage as well as reproduction, and consists of internalised schemes of perception and action common to members of the same group (Bourdieu, 1977/2013). As a multiracial and multiethnic society, Trinidad and Tobago is a melting pot of cultural practices informed by its colonial past, diasporic population and widening social disparity. As a society that continues to struggle with issues of violence, exploring solutions to violence among adolescents in a community affected by violence seems relevant to the evolving cultural identity of Trinidad and Tobago and the habitus of its adolescent youth.

Approaches to ethnographic research

Ethnography has a long-established qualitative approach to research that involves direct and sustained interactions with people in the context of their daily lives and cultures, and creates opportunities for rich descriptions, which examine and relate complex areas of inquiry. Hammersley and Atkinson (2019) reflect on the emergence of ethnography in nineteenth-century Western anthropology, where social anthropologists typically conducted ethnographic fieldwork through immersing themselves in an unfamiliar community or culture for extended periods of time, with the purpose of documenting and interpreting distinctive ways of life, belief systems and values integral to that society. This form of sociological inquiry developed alongside other approaches to ethnography that utilised observational techniques to explore the actions and experiences of marginalised rural and urban groups within Western societies (Brewer, 2000).

While the origins of ethnography are somewhat complex and shifting, Hammersley and Atkinson (2019) outline key features of ethnographic work that include the study of people's actions within the context of daily life; data gathering from multiple sources; relatively unstructured approaches to data collection, which do not implement a fixed design or interpretation at the onset; an in-depth focus via small-scale investigation; and the analysis of data through interpreting meanings, functions and consequences of actions and practices. As such, ethnography is not a specific data collection technique, but rather a multi-technique qualitative approach through which mixed methods, appropriate to a situation, can be adapted and utilised by researchers.

In practice, ethnographic fieldwork can take the form of diverse experiences with participants including, workshops, encounters, relationships, observations and conversations, in addition to documents and artefacts in physical and virtual spaces. It also involves researchers in frequent reflection on the data that is gathered and deliberation towards recognising patterns or themes as they unfurl. This inductive process enables researchers to engage with participants, and to use new and varying methods as further information or questions emerge (Parthasarathy, 2008).

Interviews are another feature of ethnographic fieldwork, where in-person encounters enable researchers to request information from participants using highly structured or semi-structured interview schedules in the form of open or closed questions (Brewer, 2000). Interviews can be used to collect verbal reports of behaviour, meanings, attitudes and feelings that are not necessarily observed in the moment but are a reflection on the information requested.

There are significant hurdles to fieldwork, however, which lie in ethically obtaining access to data. Gaining access to and recruiting potential participants typically require the support of a gatekeeper, who is able to help the researcher negotiate levels of access through building trust (O'Reilly, 2009). Negotiation and trust also play a role in determining whether research is permissible, and they guide the constraints imposed on the researcher in the field. Additionally, negotiating access to data essentially includes obtaining informed consent, respecting the privacy of participants, and being sensitive to potentially harmful consequences such as exploitation (Hammersley and Atkinson, 2019).

Participant collaboration in research facilitates a unique involvement in the knowledge-production process in a way that enables participants to engage as co-researchers and to withdraw from familiar routines, forms of interactions and power relationships, to question and rethink existing interpretations of situations (Bergold and Thomas, 2012). This enables participants to contribute to the development of approaches that might have direct benefit in their own future, thereby ensuring that marginalised groups are given opportunities to be heard and respected (Dold and Chapman, 2011; Bergold and Thomas, 2012).

Bergold and Thomas (2012) note that participatory elements in research design can support examination of the social world and habitual practice through joint collaboration that generates greater understanding and empowerment. Nevertheless, participation requires that social and political conditions are conducive to democratic processes, and that participants are afforded a safe space to disclose their perspectives and experiences. In Cheney's (2011) model of participatory ethnography, young people were involved as contributing participants in assessing the needs of orphans and vulnerable children. This approach to research facilitated a meaningful contribution to the development of insights on policy and practice with the marginalised group and initiated transformative relationships between participants and their communities. Although challenges with ethics, access and coordination emerged in practice, Cheney proposes that collaboration improved the quality of the findings through strengthened relationships among stakeholders and increased organisational commitment to children's rights.

Methodology

In my investigation into understanding how cultural arts practices might be relevant for improving the psychosocial wellbeing of adolescents affected by violence, utilising a participatory ethnography enabled me to engage in qualitative research of a complex issue that explored the perceptions and experiences of a typically marginalised group. It helped me to acknowledge the value of participants as experts in the issues directly affecting their lives and empowered them as active participants in the production of knowledge that can meaningfully contribute to the development of future interventions and policies.

My study used mixed methods of ethnographic fieldwork and semi-structured group discussions with adolescents to collect data that was guided by emerging questions and themes in informal conversation and observation. I drew from Cheney's (2011) model of participatory ethnography with vulnerable children and adopted Jeffrey and Troman's (2004) time-flexible approach to ethnography, which supported my area of inquiry and the constraints I experienced as a part-time researcher.

During the course of an academic school year, my ethnographic fieldwork with adolescents at a high school in Laventille helped me to build rapport and to collaborate with a group that engaged in discussions about the impact of violence on their psychosocial wellbeing, and the potential for cultural arts practices to offer beneficial interventions to cope with difficult experiences. Ethnographic fieldwork was conducted in the music, art and dance classes of adolescents at the school, while group discussions were held in the school library, which seemed to offer participants a safe and private space for conversation. The discussion group consisted of seven teenaged adolescents, affected by violence, who reside in a community and engage with the arts at school and in their community.

To ensure ethical practice in the collection of data, I obtained permission to access participants through the Ministry of Education and the school. Data from fieldwork and discussions were anonymised and kept confidential. Participants were provided with information outlining the research project, their roles, expectations and potential risks, which were discussed with participants and parents prior to consent. Participants were also informed of their right to withdraw from the study at any stage, without giving any reason, and the school counsellor was made available to assist participants as a measure of psychological safety. Additionally, group discussions emphasised confidentiality, anonymity and the avoidance of/procedures for the disclosure of sensitive information.

Results

The following results reflect themes elicited from data collection. Data was interpreted using thematic analysis as described by Braun and Clarke (2006).

Violence

Fieldwork and group discussions with adolescent participants reflected themes related to violence in the context of their school and their community. Violent and delinquent behaviour seemed to be entrenched in the culture of the school as normative experiences and practices. In my routine visits, I was often greeted by the presence of police cars or scenes of students receiving discipline for delinquent or violent behaviour. Delinquent behaviour included truancy, vandalism, gambling and the use of illicit substances. Discipline took the form of removal from the classroom, stern lectures by teachers, reports to parents, suspension or the intervention of police to address physical conflict and illicit activity. In instances of physical fights, teachers often intervened to deescalate or to separate students, who were then taken to the school's dean for further intervention. In group discussions, fights were considered 'normal', and participants seemed desensitised to them (Savahl et al., 2013). One participant even related, 'that is one thing it will always have in a school'.

However, there were also instances of fighting at the school that were particularly intense. During one such incident, I recorded my experience.

> *A fight has erupted in the schoolyard, just outside of the staffroom.*
> *'What the hell wrong with you!'*
> *There is a large group of students outside. I see a piece of wood is being brandished by*
> *a boy.*
> *'Fight! Fight! Fight!'*

The male teachers run outside to separate the boys. Two boys are wrestling each other just outside of the staffroom in full view of the staff. One pushes the other against the wall and the other pushes back to free himself.
Some of the female teachers come into the staffroom.
'Lock the door. I not going out there. Let them call the police and dismiss the school again.'
The teachers watch outside from the large windows. They are huddled around the doors and windows as chaos ensues outside. I can barely see what is going on, other than large groups of students crowding and running along the schoolyard. One teacher returns to the staffroom with a long iron rod. She tells the staff that she took it from a student who told her that it 'won't stop him'.
Students are running to the front of the school.

My experience of witnessing this fight at the school stirred up feelings of anxiety and fear, as it was not a usual experience for me. Although I was able to shelter safely in the staffroom, this incident highlighted the volatility of student behaviour and made me feel cautious of my safety in the school environment. As I later reflected on this incident with participants in the group, they seemed curious about my emotional response and inquired whether the fight 'seemed like a movie', or I felt 'shocked', 'disappointed', or 'frightened'.

Violence in the context of the school setting did not seem unusual to participants, and this also reflected in their views of community violence as experiences they felt 'accustomed' to. However, gang rivalry and gun violence that directly threatened their sense of safety and the safety of loved ones seemed to evoke feelings of vulnerability and helplessness. Participants seemed particularly concerned about becoming targets through their association with others or from being outdoors (Adams, Morris, and Maguire, 2018).

Star:	Only the innocent people dying … The people who them warring is not the people who dying.
Cloudy:	… They killing anybody today. Family … your family could be in thing or ain't be in thing, you get hit.
Scarlet Ibis:	Yeah, you getting hit just so.

Continual exposure to violence in the community can influence the likelihood of adolescents engaging in delinquent and aggressive behaviours (Foote, 2010). My frequent observation of fights and delinquent behaviours at the school seemed to mirror the prevalence of violence in the surrounding community. I also observed that many participants related to artistic and musical forms that explored themes of violence similar to those they experienced.

In group discussions, participants reflected on differences between the musical genres they preferred, and those taught at school. In particular, they seemed to relate to dancehall, a genre of Jamaican music that is popular among many urban youth. One participant referred to this style of music as 'gangster tune'. Jackman (2010) notes that fans of dancehall music identify with its creators, since both groups often share similarities in their socio-economic background. However, frequent references to sexual behaviours and the promotion of violence in lyrics pose concerns for the development of adolescent identities amidst influences of violence.

Visual images at the school also referenced themes of violence, at times. In my visit to one of the classrooms, I walked along a corridor that was embellished with graffiti. While many of these images stated the names of students, I also noticed that some referred to rival gangs present in the community.

On another occasion, I recall the remarks of a student as he drew a figure with guns in art class.

> *'One shot with that.'*
> *He wants to ensure the character is donned with an AK47 and offers to draw the guns for his friend.*
> *'Guns take precious time to draw.'*
> *The boy then turns toward me.*
> *'You don't know about guns?'*

This served to remind me of the wider context of the school setting, as geographically situated in an embattled community.

Psychosocial wellbeing

Savahl et al. (2013) notes that exposure to violence can lead to short-term and long-term negative psychosocial effects such as depression, anxiety, somatisation, post-traumatic stress, low self-esteem, loneliness, suicidality, sleep disturbance, emotional desensitisation and risky sexual behaviours. In group discussions, participants were invited to reflect on their understanding of wellbeing and the potential impact of violence on psychosocial wellbeing. Participants recognised that wellness encompasses a range of factors, including physical, mental, financial, emotional and social wellbeing. They explored aspects of wellbeing in relation to violence and shared that feelings of being 'hurt', 'mad', 'unsafe', 'down', suicidal and socially withdrawn might emerge when people experience loss.

Sky: Violence could am, affect, could affect, am … emotional wellbeing because if you was good with somebody for real long and thing, and you was now speaking to the person and then after you hear the person died, it go hurt you because you was there for the person and thing and next thing you know that happen.

Cloudy: And mentally … When them thing happen to me, it does affect you all how. Death and thing is a serious thing. It does make you want to go real mad.

Sky: Because you go start to go mad. Physical it could affect you physically because you could just kill yourself.

Grief and loss

The impact of violence on psychosocial wellbeing was also observed in the wider context of the school, when news reports confirmed that a student was killed in a gang-related, drive-by shooting outside of his home. In response to this experience of loss, many staff members and group participants shared about their grief, as well stories that reflected on their relationships with the deceased boy. Although I did not share a similar relationship, the student belonged to one of the classes I was observing. The revelation that I may have interacted with him at some point also resonated with me, and I felt sadness in response to his death.

Following the incident, staff members organised a public demonstration in memory of the boy, as an appeal to the community to reduce incidents of violence. There, I observed that visual arts and music were used by students to express feelings of sadness and loss. In the days preceding the death of the boy, I viewed the proliferation of graffiti in his classroom, that paid tribute to his life, friendships and the sadness felt by his peers. The walls and ceiling of his classroom bore messages such as 'rest in perfect peace', 'gone too soon', 'rest up high' and 'gone but not forgotten'. Students participated in the staff demonstration as well, chanting dancehall artiste Tommy Lee's 'Redemption Song', a song that speaks to the struggles of daily life and the hope for redemption.

Participants in the discussion group also noted similar responses to loss in their community, where people would share stories about the deceased and engage in distinctly more disruptive forms of public protest, as a means grieving and securing justice.

Sky: Yeah well everybody in the community will come and say what they will think about the person that die, or what they didn't know about the person that die.

Cloudy: What they think about … and sometimes they does protest about it. Probably not the right way but … how them feel, how them want they justice, they go block up the road, put tires in the road and you know? Burn garbage and them kind of thing. (laughs) Because if … they wouldn't get no justice out of it so them have to do them thing to get justice for them to feel better about them loss.

In discussions that followed this experience of loss, participants were encouraged to reflect on how the arts might assist their psychosocial wellbeing.

Me: … How do you think something like music would help somebody who is affected by violence?

Sunny: Listen to calm music to calm yourself … To take yourself out of that zone, you know? … You go be vex, and sometimes you does be looking through pictures and thing, you know?

They often referenced the arts as a mechanism for relaxation and escape from difficult emotions such as anger and sadness. For them, this took the form of listening to music, watching photographs or films, or engaging with movement through dance or exercise. Additionally, the arts seemed to remind them of more positive aspects of their community, particularly when they shared about the murals in their neighbourhood parks and the sounds of drumming or steel pan near their homes.

Reflection

Ethnographic fieldwork and group discussions afforded rich descriptions on the impact of violence on participants, as well as perspectives on how cultural arts can improve psychosocial wellbeing and help to convey emotions and experiences of violence. During my visits to the school, I was often confronted by a pervasive and stark reality that violence played a pivotal role in the everyday lives of adolescents. Violence seemed embedded in the culture and habitus of students and emerged in their physical expression of anger and frustration, as well as in the visual and musical art forms they created or embraced.

Simultaneously, their visceral connection with the arts enabled them to cope with vulnerable encounters with sadness, grief and loss through story-telling, graffiti, song and performative protest. In particular, their use of graffiti helped them to embody the significance of the grief they felt, while preserving their need for privacy and anonymity. Furthermore, the public demonstration and chanting they engaged with appeared to serve as type of healing ritual in that it unified them as a collective unit and gave them a sense of hope for redemption.

The arts also provided a pathway for relaxation and escape from reality, especially in the form of popular film and music, which adolescents felt had a positive effect on their mood. Likewise, the presence of cultural arts in their community refreshed their perspective of the world around them and gave them opportunities to reflect on positive memories and experiences.

In my personal reflection on this methodology of research, I noted difficulty with accessing participants and maintaining consistency in group discussions, which led to feeling frustrated with institutional processes and unsure of my ability to meaningfully engage participants. Oftentimes, I felt aware of my privilege as an outsider and observer of their experiences, and this challenged me to reflect on my ability to accurately capture the perspectives of this vulnerable group. The participatory and ethnographic nature of my research process played an important role in alleviating some of my concerns, as participant observations and contributions guided the discussions we held, provided me with direct insights into their emotions and ways of thinking, and proved useful in emerging developments at the school and in the community.

Although ethnographic studies are collected within a specific socio-cultural context, I submit that participatory approaches to qualitative research can meaningfully contribute to understanding complex issues of violence, psychosocial wellbeing and cultural arts in a manner that acknowledges the voices of those who are directly affected by the issues explored. It is also my hope that this research conveys my feeling of urgency with which greater focus can be placed on addressing violence in schools and communities through youth participation in research and involvement with the arts.

References

Adams, E.B., Morris, P.K., and Maguire, E.R. (2018) 'The impact of gangs on community life in Trinidad', *Race and Justice*, pp. 1–24. doi: 10.1177/2153368718820577

Bergold, J., and Thomas, S. (2012) 'Participatory research methods: A methodological approach in motion', *Forum Qualitative Sozialforschung*, 13(1), art. 30 [Online]. Available at: http://dx.doi.org/10.17169/fqs-13.1.1801

Bourdieu, P. (2013). 'Structures and the habitus' in: Nice, R. (trans.) *Outline of a theory of practice*. 19th edn. Cambridge University Press. (Original work published 1977).

Braun, V., and Clarke, V. (2006) 'Using thematic analysis in psychology', *Qualitative Research in Psychology*, 3(2), pp. 77–101. Available at: https://doi.org/10.1191/1478088706qp063oa

Brereton, B. (2010) 'The historical background to the culture of violence in Trinidad and Tobago', *Caribbean Review of Gender Studies: A Journal of Caribbean Perspective on Gender and Feminism*, 4, pp. 1–16. Available at: https://sta.uwi.edu/crgs/february2010/journals/BridgetBrereton.pdf

Brewer, J.D. (2000) *Ethnography*. In, Series: Understanding social research. Buckingham; Philadelphia, PA: Open University Press.

Cheney, K. (2011) 'Children as ethnographers: Reflections on the importance of participatory research in assessing orphans' needs', *Childhood*, 18(2), pp. 166–179.

Dold, C.J., and Chapman, R.A. (2011) 'Hearing a voice: Results of a participatory action research study', *Journal of Child and Family Studies*, 21(3), pp. 512–519.

Farnum, M., and Schaffer, R. (1998) *Youth arts handbook: Arts programs for youth at risk* [Online]. Available at: http://youtharts.artsusa.org/pdf/youtharts.pdf

Foote, R. (2010) *Predictors of youth aggression: An introduction*. St. Augustine, Trinidad and Tobago: UWI Open Campus.

Freytes Frey, A., and Cross, C. (2011) 'Overcoming poor youth stigmatization and invisibility through art: A participatory action research experience in Greater Buenos Aires', *Action Research*, 9(1), pp. 65–82. Available at: https://doi.org/10.1177%2F1476750310396951

Hall, S. (1996) 'Introduction: Who needs "identity"?' in Hall, S., and du Gay, P. (eds.) *Questions of cultural identity*. London: SAGE Publications. pp. 1–17.

Hall, S. (1997) 'The work of representation' in S. Hall (ed.) *Representation: Cultural representations signifying Pract*. London: SAGE Publications & The Open University Press. pp. 13–74.

Hammersley, M., and Atkinson, P. (2019) *Ethnography: Principles in practice*. London: Routledge.

Hocoy, D. (2002) 'Cross-cultural issues in art therapy', *Art Therapy - American Art Therapy Association*, 19(4), pp. 141–145. Available at: http://www.tandfonline.com/doi/pdf/10.1080/07421656.2002.10129683

Horne, L. (2003) *The evolution of modern Trinidad and Tobago*. Trinidad: Eniath's Printing Co Ltd.

Jackman, W.M. (2010) Dancehall and Hip-hop: Youth perceptions of sexuality and violence. *Caribbean Dialogue,* 15(1), pp. 27–40.

Jeffrey, B., and Troman, G. (2004) 'Time for ethnography', *British Educational Research Journal,* 30(4), pp. 535–548.

Malchiodi, C. (2014) *Breaking the silence: Art therapy with children from violent homes.* London: Routledge.

McLeod, J. (2011) *Qualitative research in counselling and psychotherapy.* London: SAGE Publications.

Office of Education and Culture/DHDEC, Executive Secretariat for Integral Development Organization of American States. (2011) *Towards a culture of non-violence: The role of arts and culture-field kit [Online].* Available at: https://www.oas.org/en/yearofculture/DOCs/manual%20campo%20ingles.pdf

Office of the Special Representative of the Secretary-General (SRSG) on Violence against Children. (2016) *Protecting children affected by armed violence in the community [Online].* Available at: https://violenceagainstchildren.un.org/sites/violenceagainstchildren.un.org/files/documents/publications/2._protecting_children_affected_by_armed_violence_in_the_community.pdf

O'Reilly, K. (2009) *Key concepts in ethnography.* London: SAGE Publications. Available at: http://dx.doi.org/10.4135/9781446268308

Ryan, S., McCree, R., and St Bernard, G. (1997) *Behind the bridge: Poverty, patronage and politics in Laventille, Trinidad.* Kingston, Jamaica: Multimedia Production Centre, School of Education, University of the West Indies.

Parthasarathy, B. (2008) *The ethnographic case study approach.* Available at: http://www.globalimpactstudy.ord/2008/07/the-ethnographic-case-study-approach/. Retrieved August 22, 2015 .

Savahl, S., Isaacs, S., Adams, S., Carels, C.Z., and September, R. (2013) 'An exploration into the impact of exposure to community violence and hope on children's perception of well-being: A South African perspective', *Child Indicators Research* 6(3), pp. 579–592.

Swartz, D. (1997) *Culture and power: The sociology of Pierre Bourdieu.* Chicago: The University of Chicago Press.

UNICEF. (2014) *United Nations Children's Fund: Hidden in plain sight: A statistical analysis of violence against children [Online].* Available at: http://files.unicef.org/publications/files/Hidden_in_plain_sight_statistical_analysis_EN_3_Sept_2014.pdf

Williams, J.H., and Van Dorn, R.A. (1999) 'Deliquency, gangs, and youth violence' in Jenson, J.M., and Howard, M.O. (eds.) *Prevention and treatment of violence in children and youth: Etiology, assessment, and recent practice innovations.* Washington, DC: NASW Press, pp. 199–225.

World Health Organization. (2017) *Global school-based student health survey [Online].* Available at: https://www.who.int/ncds/surveillance/gshs/Trinidad_and_Tobago_2017_GSHS_FS.pdf?ua=1

6

HOW PIPPO GOT TO DRIVE A PRECIOUS CAR: DANCE MOVEMENT THERAPY IN A CENTRE FOR YOUNG OFFENDERS

Maika Campo and Heidrun Panhofer

Introduction

The 'Education Centre'[1] is a level one centre that complies with the most restrictive judicial measures for young offenders. It accommodates boys from 14 to 21 years of age who are unable to comply with their sentences through probation or restorative justice by means of social services.

Without attempting to assign a formal classification of the young offenders in the centre, certain subgroups can be identified: most of the boys come from Morocco, escaping poverty and abuse. Many arrive during their childhood, looking for a dream that sometimes turns into a nightmare.

The second profile of boys includes the second generation of immigrants. Their parents mainly stem from South America, or in few cases from Africa, and have had to work hard and struggle between adapting to a new culture and longing for their own countries of origin. Busy with their fight to survive, they often leave their children on their own while they face the difficulties of integration.

The third group of children proceed from dysfunctional families where delinquency is habitual, having lived parts of their lives without parents due to imprisonment, drug problems, abandonment, death, only to name a few. In most cases, they are familiar with the governmental system which has protected them and have agreed to comply with a judicial measure as a normal part of the process of growing up.

The fourth group consists of boys from all kinds of social situations who have turned to aggression during their adolescence and directed their anger against their parents. A last and very varied group includes those with mental illness and drug problems.

This is a very simple classification and unfortunately, it is possible for a boy to belong to more than one group. However, all subgroups suffer a lack of support resulting in delinquency; often this is linked to insecure attachments or loss and separation. In many cases, trauma is another crucial common factor encountered amongst these young offenders.

The first author of this chapter, Maika, has been working there for 13 years as a community worker within a multidisciplinary team, starting her work in this institution prior to her master's degree in Dance Movement Therapy (DMT).

The training in DMT turned out to be a remarkable turning point for her method of working and made her question her role in the institution; the juvenile detention centre focuses mainly on the behaviour of the adolescents and her function mainly dealt with identifying and evaluating that behaviour. A widely used intervention in the centre is punishment in order to re-direct behaviour patterns. However, DMT looks at the individual's inner structure and attachments patterns: it allows to recapitulate early relationships and accesses pre-verbal states through the mediation in movement (Meekums, 1990; Trevarthen, 2001a).

An awareness of the importance of the intercorporeal relationship and its potential to bring about change inspired Maika to find ways of integrating the body into her work with the boys in her care from the perspective of DMT, by transforming the weekly verbal tutorials into spaces where the verbal and non-verbal could co-exist in order to re-create a secure attachment and a stronger base from which to embark.

Young offenders, attachment and physical bonding

As a community worker at the Education Centre, Maika's function mainly in-volves accompanying a minor or young boy through a period in which he fulfils a judicial sentence which has been imposed by a judge. The juvenile detention centre is quite a coercive environment which seeks to encourage the youth to take personal responsibility but also tries to provide support and trust as a basis for the formation of bonds. The former justice plan for juvenile offenders included the forming of an affective bonding relationship as one of the fundamental tools with which to work (III Plan de Justicia Juvenil, p. 65). Unfortunately, the current justice plan for young offenders no longer includes the dimension of a bonding relationship and the focus has mainly shifted to assessing and correcting the behaviour of the offenders. If the desired behaviour is not acquired, punishment is quite frequent, putting the community worker more in the role of a prison guard than a new possible attachment figure.

There are two main theories that link attachment and delinquency: Bowlby (1944) was the first to show that continual disruption of the attachment between infant and primary caregiver could result in long term cognitive, social and emotional difficulties for an individual such as delinquency, reduced intelligence, increased aggression and depression. Furthermore, attachment theory suggests that a history of insecure attachment experiences may not in itself determine mala-daptive development but may predispose to certain mental representations of at-tachment that influence emotions, cognition and behaviours in social interactions.

Hirschi (1969) conceptualised attachment as an affective bond through which children internalise conventional norms of society; strong affective ties protect against delinquent impulses; and delinquent behaviour increases if the bond to the parent is weak. Numerous sources have since confirmed that the poor quality of affectionate care in childhood is one of the major contributing factors to vulnerability in mental health and antisocial behaviour during childhood (Hoeve et al, 2012; Shonkoff et al., 2012; Siegel, 2015; Cowan et al., 2016; Atzil et al., 2018; Gilbert, 2019; Music, 2019).

Bowlby stressed the necessity of attachment behaviour throughout our lives: 'Although the possibility of change decreases with time, change continues throughout the life cycle' (1989, p. 158). The patterns established early in life have a major impact on the children's functioning, but individual experiences continue to influence the internal model of attachment. Studies on intervention defend the idea that a relationship-based treatment can allow the appropriate development to take place (Siegel, 2007, p.120) and that complementary attachments are best for achieving a secure base in psychotherapy (Marmarosh et al., 2014). More so, not only do abandonment, separation and dysfunctional relationships form part of most of our offenders' backgrounds, trauma is also very common amongst them and is mostly ignored by the centre. Some of the Educational Centre's more recent interventions have however resulted in the re-traumatisation of these young people, adding more pain in a vicious circle.

Rebuilding a secure attachment and a safe base is one of the main needs of the boys as the correction of behaviour styles only touches the tip of a huge iceberg. A Dance Movement Therapist's interventions are based on an interpersonal relationship and 'shared corporeality' or 'intercorporeality' (Merleau-Ponty, 1964, pp. 141–143).

The therapist needs to be physically available to build a new relationship with his or her patient. Just like a mother, father or caregiver, he or she can form a profound attachment through his or her feeling and thinking body; this is an approach that allows accessing very early behaviour patterns. Stern's theory of implicit relational knowing and Fuchs' (2003) concept of intracorporeal memory both underline the far-reaching effects of our early intercorporeality. Early interactions turn into implicit relational styles for the personality.

> As a result of a learning processes which are in principle comparable to the acquiring of motor skills, people later shape and enact their relationships according to the patterns they have extracted from their primary experiences (Fuchs, 2004, p. 4).

Our attachments styles be they secure, insecure or avoidant form part of our embodied personality structure, revealing our basic attitudes and relational patterns in the world. Fundamental DMT elements such as kinaesthetic empathy, mirroring and attunement, body memory, or movement metaphor are closely tied to embodied and enactive theories and have found their place in a broader scientific framework (Koch and Fischman, 2011). These valuable contributions prompted Maika to integrate the intercorporeal relationship in her work with the offenders in order to achieve physical bonding and re-build a secure attachment and safe base which involved using DMT techniques within the weekly tutorials with the boys. The proposal of 'movement tutorials' was integrated with the verbal work which had been done previously and thereafter the tutorials started to include the possibility of body work, play, improvisation, music, dance and other forms of artistic expressions (Campo, 2014). In more recent years, DMT with young offenders has also been described by a series of other studies (Payne, 1988, 2003; Smeijsters et al., 2011; Tepper-Lewis, 2019), showing an improvement of self-image, emotion regulation, self-restraint skills and appropriate expression of emotion.

Trauma

Another common feature of the young offenders in the Education Centre is the experience of trauma. Different authors have described the relationship between trauma and the high number of juvenile offenders (Widom and Maxfield, 1996; Chamberlain and Moore, 2002; Ford et al., 2007; Kerig and Becker, 2010; Dierkhising et al., 2013). Etymologically the word 'trauma' comes from the ancient Greek meaning 'wound', but when speaking about psychological wounds, trauma does not mean just another injury but rather a disruption or rupture. Van der Kolk (2015) affirms that the imprints of traumatic experiences are organised not as coherent logical narratives but in fragmented sensory and emotional traces: images, sounds and physical sensations (p. 178).

Numerous authors speak of fragmentation and the incoherent narrative of the Self from traumatic experiences (Singer and Rexhaj, 2006; Federman and Sterenfeld, 2017). Traumatic events are experiences that may not be appropriated and integrated into a meaningful context. Fisher (2014) describes how, on one hand, human beings need psychological distance from overwhelming events such as the experience of a serious accident, rape, torture or threat of death while on the other hand, disowning of the trauma results in profound alienation from the self. Traumatic memory not only includes images and narratives but also intrusive emotions, sensory phenomena, autonomic arousal and physical actions and reactions (ibid, p. 6).

According to Fuchs' (2003, 2012) categorisations of body memory, the most indelible impression in body memory is caused by trauma:

> 'Trauma withdraws from conscious recollection but remains all the more virulent in the memory of the lived body, as if it were a foreign body' (Fuchs, 2012, p. 17).

Similar situations to those of the trauma may re-evoke similar feelings and pain, fear, panic, shame and so forth, forcing the victim to re-experience similar feelings and fragments of intense images. More so, trauma survivors are vulnerable to react with irrational responses that may be irrelevant or harmful in the present, because reminders of the past may automatically activate certain neurobiological responses (Van der Kolk, 2006).

From the perspective of movement observation and analysis (Lamb, 1965; Davis, 1970, 1987, 1991; Bartenieff, 1980; Laban, 1987, 1988, 1991; North, 1990; Davis and Markus, 2006; Moore and Yamamoto, 2012) individuals who suffer physical or psychological pain tend to take screw-like positions, twisting their bodies in two opposite directions. Physical or emotional pain may literally tend to tear us apart: we not only lose grounding (De Tord and Bräuninger, 2015) but also a clear focus.

Behnke (2012, p. 83) describes traumatic body memory as 'enduring' which in German means bearing something [aushalten]as well as lasting [fortdauern). So not only does the individual go through an experience that is extremely difficult to bear, but also at the same time the effect of the experience will last and will 'make you tough', which is the Latin meaning for 'enduring.'

In patients with a history of trauma, early attachment disruptions increase the risk of developing complex trauma disorders and the presence of diverse symptoms that are not always easy to identify, understand or treat. The possibility of working from a nonverbal, embodied and intracorporeal perspective seemed to be a clear implication and a valid starting point for the young offenders in the Education Centre.

Pippo

Pippo's history of trauma was very present. The moment when he discovered the identity of his biological mother was a shock to him and all that had been a minimum of stability to him up to that moment was shaken. He had grown up within an unstable system filled with taboos and unanswered questions, hiding not only his real identity but also creating a myth of who he might be. From the beginning, his arrival at the Education Centre had been based on a betrayal: his mother had taken him to visit the place, and Pippo thought that he had to 'sign some papers' as he had on other occasions before the judge. But his mother had never informed him that he would remain in the detention centre to fulfil a one-year sentence and he was informed that he could not return to his family and that he would stay for an undefined period of time 'with us', by complete strangers.

Maika was not present at this crucial moment of his arrival but other team members presented her to the new arrival, describing him as a wild animal that had been closed up in a cage for Pippo, did not accept his detention and acted this out by punching and hitting walls and insulting and threatening staff, all of which, according to the centre's rules, were intolerable and sanctionable behaviours.

When Maika met Pippo for the first time in person, he had already been punished, locked up in his room and appeared defeated. There was no more shouting or fists, but almost nothing. The traumatic scenes following his mother's betrayal seemed to be a leitmotif in his life as Pippo had grown up believing that his grandmother was his mother. He explained to Maika that one day the woman who lived next door with her two other children (who he thought was his aunt) suddenly announced that she was his mother. This sudden discovery when he was seven years old shook his fragile sense of self. Furthermore, the introduction of the existence of a rejected father figure exacerbated his complex cultural identity of being Spanish, a Gypsy, with a French father. This threefold identity caused him considerable distress, as his father had been completely disowned by his mother's side of the family and their negative feelings towards the father consequently projected onto Pippo: 'He is just like his father'.

When Pippo arrived in the Education Centre after a series of offences, he was continuously in motion and used verbal language as his main vehicle of destruction. No psychiatric diagnosis had been undertaken to describe an insecure or avoidant attachment style or a possible attachment disorder. However, from a movement observational perspective (Davis, 1970, 1987, 1991; Bartenieff, 1980; North, 1990; Davis and Markus, 2006), Pippo was by no means present in his own body. He was pure action; quick, intense, without grounding (De Tord and Bräuninger, 2015) and had no awareness of the space around him. He would use sudden timing, no transitions and plenty of firm weight (Bartenieff, 1980; Laban, 1987, 1988, 1991; North, 1990). Just like a wild little animal, he sang, danced, shouted and gesticulated, no matter the context or the consequences. Time and space did not mean anything to him; only what was immediate made sense. This was something very evident. At the same time, his need to relate and his search for somebody that he could hold onto were obvious. He had to stop, focus and give himself time in order to do so, but he desperately needed somebody at his side. He could damage others and he damaged himself. At that point, he would stop and cry as if he were a little boy, suddenly looking for contact. This call for help was a key factor for our relationship and Maika's proposal to integrate movement into his individual weekly tutorials.

By the time the movement tutorials started, Maika and Pippo had already shared 23 verbal tutorials and their bond had been formed without having explicitly included their bodies. When starting with a verbal check-in, followed by a proper warm-up, development of the session and final check-out, which is a common framework belonging to a DMT session (Stanton Jones, 1992; Meekums, 2002; Panhofer, 2005), Pippo engaged enthusiastically. The mere fact of having been offered such a space where he could listen to music and move allowed some of Pippo's core identity to be recognised. From the beginning, he was keen to offer his 'vast movement repertoire' to his tutor, including some ballet classes he had taken when he was young, recalling and sharing 'grandes jettés' and pirouettes with her. It was clear that he confronted this new phase in his life by giving all that he had, exploring aspects of his childhood. The material he brought to therapy was expressed in the form of movement. He wanted Maika to reflect upon it and evidenced an immense need to be seen and recognised, to experiment and test out different facets of his identity.

Panksepp (1998) argues that 'affect is accompanied by the impulse to move, express, or act in some way which fulfils the function of the emotional operating system' (Panksepp, 1998, p. 18; Carroll, 2006, p. 52). Movement and emotions were a fundamental part of their interactions. Pippo never tired of showing himself and asking her to watch while he was dancing, jumping and trying to rise and fall in a playful way as if enacting his own past and future.

At the same time, Maika felt Pippo's absolute lack of boundaries and his immense need of support; in the beginning, she had to be very close to him and at times even support him physically. He had a hard time finishing his actions and his relationship with Maika was rather fusional, initiating a lot of physical and eye contact with her, and treating her with a lot of care. As his tutor, she took time to mirror his actions, attune with him and provide empathetic responses to his movement proposals. This 'execution of behaviour that expresses the character of the feelings in a shared state, without mimicking the exact behavioural expression of an inner state' (Stern, 1991, p. 177) gave Pippo a sense of being held and supported, re-constructing a secure inner base as a basis for a healthy identity.

The community workers of the centre were supportive and, Maika tried to be completely authentic with him at all times, trying to offer her body-mind (Acolin, 2016). Little by little he found his way to her, firstly by allowing himself to fall, to cry, at times to search for confrontation and to fight and express the rage he had inside, of which he had so much. Once he was able to focus; he was able to slow down his constant movement. He expressed this as the experience of allowing what came out of his mouth to pass through his heart and his head, a clear indication that something had started to connect, and his growing consciousness of this.

He became aware of the relationship that had formed with Maika but also with other community workers in the centre, leading to a feeling of integration. The shared movement space was converted into a place where he could 'feel himself feeling'.

The movement session offered continuous discovery for Pippo. From there, he started to construct his own roots, stamp with his heels, all while taking risks, falling many times and most of the times getting back up for as Eger (2018) notes, 'recovery does not have to do with recuperation, but with discovery' (Eger, 2018, p. 409).

Halfway through his juridical sentence his grandmother, the woman who had raised him died, throwing him back into a moment of crisis and bereavement. However, the quality of the bond that had been formed between him and Maika enabled him to feel emotionally held and he used the movement tutorials constructively to work through the pain of his loss.

Pippo went through a phase of depression, accompanied by a period of not needing to move. He found himself confronted with endings, the loss of his grandmother and the approaching farewell to his time in the centre, re-opening old wounds. At the penultimate tutorial, he expressed not wanting to attend, while at the same time walking to the space with his tutor. He did not want to use music, nor move. He started by saying that the world was filth and it would be best to destroy it all and start over again. Maika reminded him that this seemed a little bit like the present moment he was living, having to leave a place where he had lived for a whole year and confront a new situation where his grandmother was not present anymore. Everything was unpredictable and frightening but at the same time offering new possibilities. When Maika asked what he needed now, he answered: 'To drink a big chocolate milkshake.' She followed his game and pretended to serve two of these drinks, offering one to himself and starting to sip the other one herself. From that moment he said that he would need a Ferrari, but they'd need to pump up the wheels since they had lost air. So they put themselves to the task, creating a story in which ten years had passed, Pippo needed money, so he cast his tutor in the role of the director of the institution and negotiated with her to see if she would buy his precious car. During the final check-out, Pippo drew a whirlpool, surrounded by guns and drugs. He said that he wanted to avoid these, took time to reflect and finally added the silhouette of his own hand in the middle of it all.

His enactment seemed to reflect clearly upon the relationship(s) he had created within the centre, the Ferrari symbolising something precious that had come about for him in exchange and that he wished to acquire. He had not suggested stealing the precious car and understood that the tyres needed pumping up and that he could take care of mending the admired vehicle together with his tutor. Pippo had become conscious of the dangerous current of crime, drugs and guns that had dragged him down over the years but placing his own hand in the middle of his final drawing could be understood as an attempt to take responsibility for his actions from now on, or at least try to do so.

In his last session, Pippo enacted a dance about his identity, using verticality and strength in order to find his roots with each step while Maika assumed the role of witness. The attentive presence of a witness served to bear testimony to the diverse expressions of Pippo's identities but also significantly impacted on the quality of engagement for the dancer/mover as it enabled a level of deep attention that is less accessible without this presence (Adler, 1999, pp. 153–154). This aspect of the Mover Witness Dyad reflects the need for a 'safe space' comparable to Winnicott's (1960) 'holding environment' thus the psychological containment that the mother/witness provides for the infant/mover, by demonstrating highly focused attention and concern, is metaphorically recreated in the MWD (Meekums, 1990, p. 53).

Discussion

The Educational Centre represents repressive authority and therefore is the authoritative parent against which the sentenced, young offenders' rebel. At the same time, it is a place where they can stop, take care of themselves both physically and psychologically, and heal. So, in a unique way, it provides a 'limiting-containing' environment for their extremely risky actions and the necessary containment for the movement tutorials. There, instead of focussing on mere behavioural change, the relationship with the young person is placed at the centre as the main tool to promote change (Siegel, 2007). Pippo, as with so many others in the institution, arrived with a sad story of betrayal and abandonment and presented insecure attachment behaviour. Enduring traumatic situations had toughened his behaviour and converted him, in some ways, into a wild animal fighting for survival. The relationship created throughout the movement tutorials offered him primarily the experience of a reliable adult who was available physically and emotionally in order to witness his process of change.

The setting of the Education Centre, though not primarily therapeutic, provided Maika with the opportunity to offer an alternative life experience, but above all, the possibility to respond to Pippo's actions, providing emotional attunement which he had been badly lacking throughout his childhood.

During the movement tutorials, Pippo became increasingly aware of his movements and overwhelming emotions. This allowed him to recall and re-experience his insecure and avoidant relational patterns, which had been formed by abandonment, loss and betrayal. Consideration and involvement of the body and its expression offered a more comprehensive picture of his story and allowed Pippo to respond, beyond a purely cognitive level. Bodywork, movement, play, improvisation and dance allowed access to preverbal stages and unconscious relational patterns. In a creative, playful way they were able to recapitulate his early relationships and mediate some of his traumatic experiences in movement (Meekums, 1990; Trevarthen, 2001b), re-formulating a secure basis and stable attachment figures. Recent findings from attachment neurobiology (Schore, 2014) describe the involvement of primarily right-side brain activities when it comes to forming an attachment, supporting thus the need of the integration of an implicit – at times – unconscious and corporeal approach in order to promote change.

Conclusion

Abandonment, separation and dysfunctional relationships, as well as trauma, form part of most of the offenders' backgrounds in the Education Centre. The connection between these factors and juvenile crime has been largely described (Bowlby, 1944; Hirschi, 1969; Hoeve et al, 2012; Shonkoff et al., 2012; Siegel, 2015; Cowan et al., 2016; Atzil et al., 2018; Gilbert, 2019; Music, 2019).

DMT as an embodied and enactive form of psychotherapy (Koch and Fischman, 2011) deals very directly with the individual's inner structure and attachment patterns and allows the recapitulation of early relationships and access pre-verbal states through movement (Meekums, 1990; Trevarthen, 2001a). Advances in psychotherapy have equally shifted to a relational 'two-person psychology' approach, placing the relationship at the centre of attention in order to promote change, beyond mere behavioural changes.

Additional studies are certainly needed to fully understand how the client and therapist attachment dimensions influence the psychotherapy process and what facilitates a secure base in treatment. However, building on several decades of attachment theory research and in the light of the recent advances in neuroscience, it remains clear that the dimension of a bonding relationship must be central in the work with young offenders. This chapter proposes the integration of the body in order to work on early stages of human development, to re-create new secure attachments and overcome trauma and loss in order to break the vicious circle of juvenile crime.

Note

1 All names have been anonymised.

References

Acolin, J. (2016) 'The mind–body connection in dance/movement therapy: Theory and empirical support'. *American Journal on Dance Therapy,* 38, pp. 311–333. Available at: https://doi.org/10.1007/s10465-016-9222-4. (Accessed: 22 July 2020)

Adler, J. (1999) 'Who is the witness? A description of authentic movement', in Pallaro, P. (ed.) *Authentic movement. Essays by Mary Starks Whitehouse, Janet Adler and Joan Chodorow.* Philadelphia: Jessica Kingsley Publishers, pp. 141–159.

Atzil, S., Gao, W., Fradkin, I., and Barrett, L.F. (2018) 'Growing a social brain', *Nature Human Behaviour,* 2, pp. 624–636.

Bartenieff, I. (1980) *Body movement: Coping with the environment.* New York: Gordon & Breach.

Behnke, E.A. (2012) 'Enduring: A phenomenological investigation', in Koch, S., Fuchs, T., Summa, M., and Müller, C. (eds.) *Body memory, metaphor and movement.* Amsterdam: John Benjamins.

Bowlby, J. (1944) Forty-four juvenile thieves: Their characters and home life. *International Journal of Psychoanalysis,* 25(19-52), pp. 107–127.

Bowlby, J. (1989) *Una base segura. Aplicaciones clínicas de una teoría del apego.* Barcelona: Editorial Paidós Ibérica S.A.

Campo, M. (2014) 'Una tutoría en movimiento en el Centro Educativo Ibaiondo', in En Panhofer, H., and Ratés, A. (eds.) *Encontrar, compartir, aprender. Máster en Danza Movimiento Terapia. Jornadas del 10° aniversario.* Barcelona: Servei de Publicacions. Universitat Autónoma de Barcelona, pp. 179–186.

Carroll, R. (2006) 'A new era for psychotherapy', in Corrigall, J., Payne, H., and Wilkinson, H. (eds.) *About a body. Working with the embodied mind in psychotherapy.* East Sussex: Editorial Routledge, pp. 50–62.

Chamberlain, P., and Moore, K.J. (2002) 'Chaos and trauma in the lives of adolescent females with antisocial behavior and delinquency', *Journal of Aggression, Maltreatment Trauma,* 6(1), pp. 79–108.

Cowan, C.S.M., Callaghan, B.L., Kan, J.M., and Richardson, R. (2016) 'The lasting impact of early-life adversity on individuals and their descendants: Potential mechanisms and hope for intervention', *Genes, Brain and Behavior,* 15(1), pp. 155–168. Available at: https://doi.org/10.1111/gbb.12263. (Accessed: 23 August 2020)

Davis, M. (1970) 'Movement characteristics of hospitalized psychiatric patients'. Proceedings of Fifth Annual Conference of the American Dance Therapy Association, pp. 25–45.

Davis, M. (1987) 'Steps to achieving observer agreement: The LIMS reliability project', Movement Studies, 2, pp. 7–19.

Davis, M. (1991) 'Guide to movement analysis methods part 2: Movement Psychodiagnostic Inventory'. Unpublished manual.

Davis, M., and Markus, K. (2006) 'Misleading cues, misplaced confidence: An analysis of deception detection patterns', *American Journal on Dance Therapy*, 28(2), Fall/Winter, pp. 107–126.

De Tord, P., and Bräuninger, I. (April 2015) 'Grounding: Theoretical application and practice in dance movement therapy', *Arts Psychotherapy*, 43, pp. 16–22. Available at: http://dx.doi.org/10.1016/j.aip.2015.02.001 (Accessed: 23 August 2020)

Dierkhising, C.B., Ko, S.J., Woods-Jaeger, B., Briggs, E.C., Lee, R., and Pynoos, R.S. (2013) 'Trauma histories among justice-involved youth: findings from the National Child Traumatic Stress Network', *European Journal of Psychotraumatology*, 4, 10.3402/ejpt.v4i0.20274. https://doi.org/10.3402/ejpt.v4i0.20274 (Accessed: 23 August 2020)

Eger, E. (2018) *La bailarina de Auschwitz*. Barcelona: Editorial Planeta.

Federman, D.J., and Sterenfeld, G.Z. (2017) 'Overcoming trauma. When verbal language is not enough' in Payne, H. (ed.) *Essentials of dance Movement Psychotherapy. International perspectives on theory, research and practice*. London: Editorial Routledge, pp. 171–184.

Fisher, J. (2014) 'Putting the pieces together: 25 years of learning trauma treatment', *Psychotherapy Networker*, May/June, 2014, pp. 1–21. Available at: https://janinafisher.com/pdfs/twenty-five-years.pdf, (Accessed: 23 August 2020)

Fromm, E. (1991) *Del tener al ser*. Barcelona: Editorial Paidós.

Fuchs, T. (2003) 'The memory of the body', unpublished manuscript [Online]. Available at: http://www.klinikum.uniheidelberg.de/fileadmin/zpm/psychatrie/ppp2004/manuskript/fuchs.pdf (Accessed: 8 December 2019)

Fuchs, T. (2004) 'Neurobiology and psychotherapy: An emerging dialogue', *Current Opinion in Psychiatry*, 17(6), pp. 479–485.

Fuchs, T. (2012) 'The phenomenology of body memory' in Koch, S., Fuchs, T., Summa, M., and Müller, C. (eds.) *Body memory, metaphor and movement*. Amsterdam: John Benjamins.

Ford, J.D., Chapman, J.F., Hawker, J., and Albert, D. (2007) *Trauma among youth in the juvenile justice system: Critical issues and new directions*. National Center for Mental Health and Juvenile Justice. Available at: http://www.ncjrs.gov/App/publications/abstract.aspx?ID=254218 (Accessed: 23 August 2020).

Gilbert, F. (2019) 'Psychotherapy for the 21st century: An integrative, evolutionary, contextual, biopsychosocial approach', *Psychology and Psychotherapy: Theory, Research and Practice*, 92(2), pp. 164–189. Available at: https://doi.org/10.1111/papt.12226 (Accessed: 23 August 2020)

Hirschi, T. (1969) *Causes of delinquency*. Berkeley, CA: University of California Press.

Hoeve, M., Stams, G.J.L., Van der Put, C.E., Semon Dubas, J., Van der Laans, P.H., and Gerris, J.R.M. (2012) 'A meta-analysis of attachment to parents and delinquency', *Journal of Abnormal Child Psychology*, 40, pp. 771–785. doi: 10.1007/s10802-011-9608-1

III plan de Justicia Juvenil en la Comunidad Autónoma de Euskadi 2008–2012. (2009) *Vitoria-Gasteiz: Editorial Eusko Jaurlaritzaren Argitalpen Zerbitzu Nagusia* [Online]. Available at: https://www.euskadi.eus/contenidos/plan/iii_plan_pjj_2008_2012/es_iii_pjj/adjuntos/III%20Plan%20Justicia%20Juvenil%2008-12.pdf (Accessed: 23 August 2020)

IV plan de Justicia Juvenil en la Comunidad Autónoma de Euskadi 2014–2018. (2015) *Vitoria Gasteiz* [Online]. Available at: https://www.irekia.euskadi.eus/uploads/attachments/6934/PLAN_JUSTICIA_JUVENIL_2014–2018_(CAST).pdf?1442911407 (Accessed: 23 August 2020)

Kerig, P.K., and Becker, S.P. (2010) 'From internalizing to externalizing: Theoretical models of the processes linking PTSD to juvenile delinquency', in Egan, S.J. (ed.) *Posttraumatic stress disorder (PTSD): Causes, symptoms and treatment*. Hauppauge, NY: Nova Science, pp. 33–78.

Koch, S., and Fischman, D. (2011) 'An embodied enactive approach to dance/movement therapy', *American Journal on Dance Therapy*, 33(1), pp. 57–72. doi: 10.1007/s10465-011-9108-4

Laban, R. (1987) *El Dominio del Movimiento*. Madrid: Ed Fundamentos.

Laban, R. (1988) *Die Kunst der Bewegung*. Wilhelmshaven: Heinrichshofen Verlag.

Laban, R. (1991) *La Danza Educativa Moderna*. Méjico: Ed Paidós.

Lamb, W. (1965) *Posture and gesture*. London: Duckworth.

Marmarosh, C.L., Kivlighan, D.M., Jr., Bieri, K., LaFauci Schutt, J.M., Barone, C., and Choi, J. (2014) 'The insecure psychotherapy base: Using client and therapist attachment styles to understand the early alliance', *Psychotherapy*, 51(3), 404–412. Available at: https://doi.org/10.1037/a0031989 (Accessed: 23 August 2020)

McLeod, S. (2015) 'The ethos of the mover/ witness dyad: an experimental frame for participatory performance', *Brolga: An Australian Journal about Dance*, 40, pp. 57–72. Available at: http://search.ebscohost.com/login.aspx?direct=true&db=ibh&AN=117067802&site=eds-live (Accessed: 23 August 2020)

Meekums, B. (1990) 'Dance movement therapy and the development of mother–child interaction', M.Phil. thesis. University of Manchester.

Meekums, B. (2002) *Creative therapies in practice: Dance movement therapy*. London: SAGE Publications.

Merleau-Ponty, M. (1964) *The primacy of perception: And other essays on phenomenological psychology, the philosophy of art, history and politics (studies in phenomenology and existential philosophy)*, Chapter 2 (trans. James. M. Edie). Evanston, IL: Northwestern University Press. pp. 12–43.

Moore, C.L., and Yamamoto, K. (2012) *Beyond words: Movement observation and analysis*. London: Routledge.

Music, G. (2019) *Nurturing children: From trauma to growth using attachment theory, psycho-analysis and neurobiology*. London, UK: Routledge.

North, M. (1990) *Personality assessment through movement*. Plymouth: Northcote House Publishers Ltd.

Panhofer, H. (2005) *El cuerpo en psicoterapia. La teoría y práctica de la Danza Movimiento Terapia*. Barcelona: Gedisa.

Panksepp, J. (1998) *Affective neuroscience: The foundations of human and animal emotions*. New York: Oxford University Press.

Payne, H. (1988) 'The use of DMT with troubled youth', in Schaefer, C. (ed.) *Innovative interventions in childcare and adolescent therapy*. London: Wiley, pp. 30–60.

Payne, H. (2003) *Dance movement therapy: Theory and practice*. London: Routledge.

Schore, A. (2014) 'The right brain is dominant in psychotherapy', *Psychotherapy*, 51(3), 388–397. Available at: http://dx.doi.org/10.1037/a0037083

Shonkoff, J.P. et al. (January 2012) 'The lifelong effects of early childhood adversity and toxic stress', *Pediatrics*, 129(1), 232–246. doi: 10.1542/peds.2011-2663

Siegel, D.J. (2007) *La mente en desarrollo. Cómo interactúan las relaciones y el cerebro para modelar nuestro ser*. Bilbao: Editorial Desclée de Brouwer S.A.

Siegel, D.J. (2015) *The developing mind: How relationships and the brain interact to shape who we are*. New York: Guilford Publications.

Singer, J.A., and Rexhaj, B. (2006) 'Narrative coherence and psychotherapy: A commentary', *Journal of Constructivist Psychology*, 19(2), pp. 209–217.

Smeijsters, H., Kil, J., Kurstjens, H., Welten, J., and Willemars, G. (2011) 'Arts therapies for young offenders in secure care: A practice-based research', *Arts Psychotherapy*, 38, pp. 41–51.

Stanton Jones, K. (1992) *Dance movement therapy in psychiatry*. London: Routledge.

Stern, D.N. (1991) *El mundo interpersonal del infante. Una perspectiva desde el psicoanálisis y la psicología evolutiva*. Buenos Aires: Editorial Paidós.

Tepper-Lewis, C. (2019) 'Description and evaluation of a dance/movement therapy programme with incarcerated adolescent males', *Body Movement and Dance in Psychotherapy*, 14(3), pp. 159–176.

Trevarthen, C. (2001a) 'Setting the scene: A window into childhood', Lecture given to the 7th professional conference of the UK Council for Psychotherapy: Revolutionary Connections Psychotherapy and Neuroscience, 7–9 September, Warwick University.

Trevarthen, C. (2001b) 'Intrinsic motives for companionship in understanding: Their origin, development, and significance for infant mental health', *Infant Mental Health Journal*, 22 (1-2, January), pp. 95–131. https://doi.org/10.1002/1097-0355(200101/04) 22:1%3C95::AID-IMHJ4%3E3.0.CO;2-6

Van der Kolk, B.A. (2006) 'Clinical implications of neuroscience research for treatment of PTSD', *New York Academy of Sciences*, pp. 1–17. doi: 10.1196/annals.1364.022

Van der Kolk, B.A. (2015) *The body keeps the score. Brain, mind and body in the healing of trauma*. New York: Editorial penguin books.

Widom, C.S., and Maxfield, M.G. (1996) 'A prospective examination of risk for violence among abused and neglected children', *Annals New York Academy of Sciences* 749, pp. 224–236.

Winnicott, D. (1960) 'The theory of the parent–child relationship', *International Journal of Psychoanalysis*, 41, pp. 585–595.

7

FROM EMPTINESS TO SYMBOL: RESEARCHING THE CONGENITALLY YOUNG BLIND CHILD IN MUSIC THERAPY

Heike Wrogemann-Becker

Introduction

Congenital blindness can severely impair the cognitive, emotional and sensorimotor development of children alongside curtailing their vital relationships with sighted carers (Fraiberg, 1977a, 1977b, 1979; Warren, 1984). Yet, the mental health of children born blind has received varying degrees of interest and neglect in psychotherapy practice and research, and likewise in the arts therapies. As a music therapist, though concerned with the phenomena of sound, I am nonetheless a very visual person. When visiting the music therapist Andreas Stark at the Hanover State Training Centre for the Blind, I was impressed by his work and by the clientele. I became curious about the intricacies of music therapy with blind children and how they could be conceptualised within my own psychodynamic frame of reference. I decided on investigating this field in my doctoral research at Hamburg University and this chapter is an abbreviated map of my findings, deliberations and conclusions.

Investigating a case cohort of six congenitally blind children aged between two-and-a-half to five years in individual music therapy sessions, the chapter describes and theorises how music therapy can enhance blind children's delayed ego-functions, and their ability to relate, interact and symbolise.

Background of the investigation: literature on blind children's psychological development

Trying to establish the background of my research, I found clusters of literature from various professional angles working with the congenitally blind; the most prominent ones came from psychology and the psychodynamic psychotherapies, especially psychoanalysis and music therapy. In the following section, I will briefly review these portions of the literature and highlight key findings.

1. Psychoanalysis and the development of congenitally blind children

Summarising psychological, psychotherapeutic and psychoanalytic papers and studies on blindness and early childhood development, Warren (1984) outlines that blindness was a particular concern in psychoanalysis in the UK and US. Numerous authors were concerned with the question how being blind from birth impacts human psychological development. Especially the American psychoanalyst Selma Fraiberg and her team found that with congenitally blind children, the beginnings of interpersonal communications, object permanence and the ensuing ability to form mental object representations were considerably lagging behind compared to sighted children. The congenitally blind child is surrounded by a world of fragments, that is, suddenly appearing and disappearing sounds, or by bouncing into physical objects whose presence could not be anticipated. In the blind child, the experience of the 'unstable' presence of objects and persons, who may materialise and disappear in an equally unpredictable and 'unforeseeable' fashion, leads to frustration and a poorly developed sense of object permanence, if not fragmentation of the object's internal representation (Fraiberg and Freedman, 1964; Fraiberg, Siegel, and Gibson, 1966; Fraiberg, 1968, 1969, 1971, 1977a, 1977b, 1979; Fraiberg and Adelson, 1973). Hence, Fraiberg and Freedman (1964), as later Dorothy Burlingham (1965), observed that especially ego development and concept formation were delayed in their blind subjects.

Based on Stern's (1990) developmental steps in sighted children's pre-verbal and verbal phase, Gruber and Hammer (2002) summarise the developmental phases of the congenitally blind child and detail which phase can or cannot be successfully completed due to the specifics of the visual impairment. Some developmental delays can thus be seen as a 'natural' development based on the conditions of the visual impairment. However, blind children, they point out, are at a huge disadvantage when it comes to intersubjective relationship formation and understanding social interactions at large. They have difficulties with understanding intentional and demonstrative gestures or augmenting their auditory percepts with additional information, that is, on the mother's face. This has grave consequence, that is, in the absence of additional visual cues, blind distressed infants mistake the mirroring and soothing sounds of their mothers as a sign that the mother, herself, is unhappy. This creates problems with the regulation of affect.

Another key concern in psychoanalytic papers on congenitally blind children has been their difficulties with symbolisation (Burlingham, 1961; Wills, 1965, 1968, 1979a, 1979b, 1981; Fraiberg and Adelson, 1973). Bishop, Hobson and Lee (2005) summarise these and several other studies and find conflicting reports about the question of symbolisation in children born blind. In their study, they found that the more socially able children fared far better with symbolisation than those with low social abilities and offer this as an explanation for differing study results. Thus, there seems to be an indication that symbolisation in blind children may depend on their successful relationships with their sighted carers.

2. Psychoanalytic positions on fragmentation and symbolisation

While psychoanalytic papers on blindness have provided useful observations and insights, other papers from the same school of thought, though not being concerned with the conditions of blindness, must be considered and are, I propose, helpful to further clarify the exact nature of the problems the blind child is struggling with.

For sighted children, Bion (1962a, 1962b) speaks of how their bodily processes gradually develop into representations and psychic contents. The infant has pre-conceptions, which turn into concepts when something that the infant expects actually happens. Initially, the infant experiences sensory percepts as meaningless or threatening 'fragments', which Bion terms 'beta elements'. These fragments can, through containment by the mother, be turned into useful psychic content, which Bion calls 'alpha elements'. These alpha elements become eventually available to the child's developing psyche through the mother's initial verbalisation.

Speaking of symbolisation, Lorenzer (1970) suggests that early mother–child interactions initially are sensory and by the specific way the mother reacts to them these interactions become sensory-*symbolic* forms. Everything that has become excluded from the symbolic and is therefore not yet understood can be apprehended in the therapeutic encounter by looking at the *scene* that unfolds between patient and therapist. It is only when looking at this entire scene, Lorenzer believes that human action can be properly understood as symbolic. Lorenzer's thoughts on the symbolic as revealed in a *scene* that can be watched, heard and felt are important as they tie in with similar thoughts by the philosopher Susanne Langer (1992), showing that both authors are highly relevant for the arts therapies. Langer suggests two distinct symbolic systems, only one of which is directly tied to language: everything represented in verbal language can be considered 'discursive' symbolism, which functions along linear, consecutive and abstract lines. On the other hand, Langer calls everything that is capable of conveying its content by presenting itself, that is, as an artistic form in art, music, drama and so forth, 'presentative' symbolism, in which content and form are inextricably perceived and understood as one.

Music therapy, as all arts therapies, greatly relies on the particular properties of what Langer calls 'presentative symbolism' which may be enriched, framed and extrapolated by the verbal, making for a happy marriage between Langer's two symbolic concepts. The question now arises whether music therapy has been applied to congenitally blind children, and if so, to which results.

Music therapy with blind children

Most papers on music therapy with the blind seem to be written from an educational or rehabilitative perspective, and only a few psychodynamic allusions can be found in some of them. Codding (2000) has systematically collected and listed papers on music therapy with blind and severely visually impaired people from 1940 to 2000 and summarises in which way music therapy was used to support, stimulate and structure the learning abilities, motory, social and verbal abilities of visually impaired children. She finds that the studies on music therapy as applied to blind children and adults were generally scarce; in most studies on music therapy and blindness, 'the primary uses of music were as *structured activity* where music was used either as structure for the assessment, or to structure non-musical learning outcomes. When music was used as a *stimulus cue or prompt*, it served as an auditory cue for spatial awareness and travel…Music was also used as a *contingency* to establish, maintain, or eliminate inappropriate non-musical behavior, or as a desirable response *incompatible* with destructive or nonproductive behavior' (188).

Orff (1982), describing an individual case, generally highlights the importance of the acoustic phenomenon and the pre-melodic play for the development of a blind girl. Kern (2006a, 2006b) shows how blind children can be supported in their wish to connect and learn, that is, enhancing their ability to orientate through sound parcours. Using a psychodynamic frame of reference and focussing on the development of contact and the relationship, Aepkers and Stark (2005) describe a six-week section of a music therapy process of several years with a 14-year-old blind boy. They stress the particular benefits of body contact and the imitation of vitality affects, as the patient's need to feel safe could not be fulfilled visually in the absence of sight and the visual gaze.

Similarly, Aepkers (2008) describes several vignettes of music therapy with nine blind patients aged 9–19 years, eight of them with an added developmental delay, and he reiterates his earlier notion of the usefulness of physical contact and highlights the importance of responding to clients' current needs emerging in therapy.

Metell (2015) researches how music therapy and its interactions can contribute to the early interaction and bonding between children with visual impairment and the sighted caregivers. Selecting and analysing moments of positive interactions in music and triangulating these with views from caregivers, she finds that music therapy enhances positive bonding patterns and early interaction. Based on these findings, she argues here, as in a later paper (2017), for a stronger link between disability studies and community music therapy.

Summary

The literature review reveals a heightened interest in the phenomenon of congenital blindness in psychoanalysis resulting in observations and some research, particularly in the 1960s and 1970s. In music therapy, as already stated by Codding (2000), there is a general scarceness of research or papers on practice or research with the blind and visually impaired; among the existing papers, many come from an educational perspective and few seem psychodynamically informed. Music therapy, as it was understood in these educational papers, sets out to change clearly defined behavioural problems in these children. Among the few papers with a psychodynamic framework, the questions of the role of music for blind children's ego development, their ability to symbolise and a systematic scrutiny of interactional forms and scenes in which such developments might be set, remain by and large unclear. Theories on symbolisation such as Bion's or Lorenzer's have yet not been considered and integrated into music therapy positions when working with blindness.

Against the backdrop of these findings from the literature, I developed my research questions:

Research questions

- In which way can music therapy be helpful for the blind children's ego development?
- Which role can music play in enhancing ego development, that is, what kinds of interactional forms can be observed? Which kinds of scenes do occur?
- Can symbolisation be observed in the investigated music therapy sessions, and if so, under which conditions?

Outline of research design and methods

Recruitment and setting

As I did not operate from a music therapy base within an institution, I needed to arrange contacts through a state school for the blind in Germany, supporting my research project. Eventually I had been assigned five congenitally blind children whose parents agreed for their child to participate, and in one case, the parents, who had heard of the project by word of mouth and had contacted me, directly referred one child.

I thus ended up with a cohort of six congenitally blind children, four girls and two boys, aged between three and seven. Out of these six, three children had added learning disabilities.

The music therapy part of my research lasted for 20–24 months, each child attending individual fortnightly non-directive music therapy sessions of 40 minutes' duration. The children's parents were not present. I saw five children in their homes for music therapy, while one attended sessions in my private practice.

Data collection

I held 201 individual sessions in total, all of which were documented in written session reports. Also, I documented five individual sessions by sound and ten by video. I hoped that that these video- and audio-tapes would enable me to see, by close comparison, if changes of interactive and musical patterns occurred that had gone unnoticed during the session, and that such recorded material might go beyond my personal description and reflection in my notes. As this material was an additional source, it enabled me to scrutinise the child and myself in interaction and to witness my own interventions.

As another source of information I wrote 40 research journals with observations and first or second thoughts on the case material as time progressed. These, I thought, would not only provide an aide-memoir to augment my case notes and my memory when eventually evaluating my material. These research journals constituted a separate set of information to triangulate and critically reflect on my own thinking, especially given the fact that I was a sole researcher investigating my own practice.

My Ph.D. supervisor oversaw my research and I regularly presented in a research group of other Ph.D. students. Also, I discussed my practice and emerging thoughts with an art psychotherapist who was similarly involved in a Ph.D. on his practice with congenitally blind children.

Method

Given the sparseness of specific literature on young congenitally blind children in music therapy, this investigation was about doing groundwork in trying to understand some of the fundamentals in musical symbol formation and apply systematic scrutiny and thought to the phenomena I encountered in my work with these children. What I was interested in was to compare and cross-reference between individual cases and arrive at some coherent underlying principles.

Following this interest, that is, comparing data from practice and gradually allowing theory formation to emerge from this process, I felt that grounded theory, as developed by Glaser and Strauss (1967/2005), would be particularly conducive to my research as a method. According to McLeod (2003), grounded theory, as an 'inductive approach', is set on developing a theory or a model, 'beginning with descriptive data and subjecting the material to increasing levels of conceptualization' (McLeod, 88). From these data, the researcher forms categories towards a 'grounded model', which is achieved by 'axial coding', a process that comprises 'looking for the linkages and connections between categories of experience' (89). Categories, as Glaser and Strauss describe, may only emerge over time from the raw data, may be changed or discarded for more useful and precise ones and eventually will be reduced to form a coherent model or theory. To elevate this process of theory building to a higher level, as Glaser and Strauss underscore, a researcher should allow other studies, which refer to the same *theoretical* problem, to influence one's work, regardless of the fact if their actual *subject* content matches the pursued study. In my case, I took this as a confirmation of my initial conception that Lorenzer's and especially Bion's theories on symbolisation, even though they do not refer to the problem of blindness, are nonetheless crucially important to understand the material of my current investigation.

Based on this thinking, I arrived at a set of research steps:

Research steps

1. Contacting the school for the blind and forming a cohort of six young blind children, obtaining permission for research and allocating a time frame to each individual child. This involved meeting the parents, explaining about the reasons for the research, laying out rules of confidentiality and data protection, and also regular exchange with parents.

2. Conducting and documenting individual non-directive music therapy sessions of 40 minutes' duration with the six children. In sessions, I always offered the same array of musical instruments: a keyboard, placed prominently in front of us, which became the main instrument that we referred to; and a basket with various small instruments, or small objects, producing sounds or offering tactile sensations. Documentation involved writing detailed session notes, describing the sessions' musical content and development, child–therapist interaction, reflection on the transference relationship, changes of musical and interactive patterns and possibly symbol formation. Also, I would use material from audio- or video-taped sessions to establish changes and developments by comparison.

3. Keeping a research journal throughout the entire process of sessions and evaluating the material as a means for reflection and triangulation.

4. Using grounded theory to scrutinise the material, trying to identify steps of development, describe and conceptualise them. Such categories would gradually emerge from the material by a flow of comparisons, descriptions and the eventual reduction of categories. This was aided by drawing mind-maps of categories and their interrelations.

5. Writing up the entire study and reflecting on my findings against the backdrop of literature from psychoanalysis and music therapy.

6. Reflecting on the process of research, the usefulness of its methodologies unexpected findings and identifying areas for future research.

Findings

For most music therapy sessions, the keyboard, placed on the floor for easy access and not requiring to be held in one's hands, served as the main instrument, with an added choice of small instruments and objects. Comparing cases I found that children initially did not explore or use the keyboard or the other instruments and objects, but only gradually did so when prompted. Only one boy had a previous knowledge of the keyboard and used it from the start. As sessions progressed, I would introduce instruments when musical stories evolved which invited the use of other objects beyond the keyboard. Over time, patterns evolved which could be described and conceptualised as separate and consecutive developmental phases of musical interaction, relationship building and symbolisation.

Developmental phase 1: from nameless forms to sequential chains: the emergence of expectation

In this initial phase, I could observe how symbolisation developed from the children's expectation of an acoustic phenomenon and the realisation of the anticipated sound. I would initially instigate these early sounds; a bit later in the process the blind children would begin to anticipate or preconceive them and finally initiate such sounds themselves.

The emergence of an expectation that eventually becomes fulfilled developed in consecutive, discernible steps and would involve the following:

1. A contact between blind child and music therapist is established.
2. The child gradually discriminates 'me' and 'not-me', including the occasional playful refusal of body contact or the therapist's involvement in musical play.
3. The child claims her or his part of the enacted scene adding the dimension of the 'third'.
4. The beginning and ending of sounds facilitates children's experience of how time is turned into musical space.

From these steps, the children became able to develop expectations or preconceptions that would eventually become real and manifest.

Summarising my insights from this initial phase, I suggest that in my therapeutic interventions, it was crucial to offer a meaning – as verbal or musical – narrative to the child's numerous scattered individual sensory percepts so that the child could not only notice them, but move towards their multimodal sensory integration.

Developmental phase 2: from fragments towards forming rhythmic trajectories

In this second developmental phase emerging from the case material, the child and I were faced with the need to organise elements that seemed fragmented and disconnected. This would often manifest as the children's agitated physical movements or as repetitive, disconnected words or babble. I responded to the children's disconnected *movement* by vocal mirroring. I took this one step further by containing the children's movements in a rhythm and a song, thus initiating and nurturing the child's ability to symbolise.

As a response to the fragmented *words* that the children produced in the sessions I was initially confused as to their 'meaning' or placement in our relationship and resolved to collect them in a notebook; this was initially of more relevance to me than to the children, as these 'floating' verbal fragments made me think of 'elements' in need of a 'container'. This written containment kept my presence, my thinking and my feeling intact in the face of the seemingly fragmented, unrelated and meaningless utterances from the children, which I understood as their response to percepts they could not mentally organise due to their sensory impairment.

However, my containment of their words by writing seemed also helpful for the children: they would leave the sessions in a surprisingly heightened sense of interpersonal awareness – and for the first time would say a personal good-bye to me acknowledging my name by the end of the sessions.

I also realised that a crucial part of this phase was that the blind child could temporarily forget my presence; here, the child was momentarily freed from the onerous tasks of intersubjectivity and from memorising me as the 'other' while my silent presence was still forming a backdrop to the therapeutic scene.

Another variation of dealing with fragments was the children's repetitive and playful regurgitating of the 'indigestible'. It came about when the children discovered by accident that one button on my keyboard produced the sound of a person being sick. This acoustic function soon became very popular was expected and sought for by the children and developed into a play. One child in particular repeatedly assigned me the role of a very unlucky mother/therapist: the child would announce feeling sick, then would continuously press the notorious 'sick' button and decidedly would always have me arrive too late with bucket, announcing that I had unfortunately 'missed it.' This was not only a source of great glee for all children, but also enabled us to construe a narrative for a fragmented psychic content that the children felt unable to process emotionally and cognitively. At a first glance, and taking the emerging story literally, it may seem that the child's 'sick' was not contained by the imaginary bucket – but nonetheless it was very well contained in the narrative and in our continuous laughing which clearly framed the situation in an 'as if' mode and therefore as symbolic.

Summarising my insights from this second developmental phase, I suggest that whatever perceptual fragments the blind child's ego could not organise, the child tried to evacuate as fragments: unrelated movements, words or vocalisations. Such fragments could gradually become organised and contained by several means: in the chains of sounds that, among many other characteristics, are the nature of song; in the pages of my notebook; and in the symbolic narrative of our musical play, that is, with the 'sick-button'.

Developmental phase 3: from rhythm towards the world of stories – Symbolisation of 'emptiness'

While the 'sick' button and its related story constituted a first symbolic narrative, it also represented a limited one: it would always run the same course, never to change or to expand. However, a more liberal use of sound, pause or absence of sound and narrative emerged in the third developmental phase: here, the children and I expanded and refined musical and verbal narratives; we formed rhythms into songs and stories. Such narratives became richer and with this enhancement the children became more actively involved in instigating, forming, expounding and limiting our musical interactions. A note or a sound may be the first thing coming to mind when we think of music. But the absence of sound, the pause or the 'silence', is, looking closely, equally important. Silence had already played a role in the second phase as it was part of the sound chains, or the space between contained fragments. Now, in the third phase, the absence of sound and the role of the pause, actively initiated by the children, became much more pronounced.

One boy in particular had honed this to perfection; he had discovered how to turn off the keyboard sound without shutting it down completely. Thus, he had the power to reduce my musical contributions or interventions to the mere clicking sound of my fingers on the keys, while totally eliminating the melody. He thus became the master of the story, of sound and of silence. At the time, I was aware that in this process and through his partly disabling actions, the boy assigned me a personal experience of disability (beingmute and ineffective) and allowed me to catch a glimpse of his world, while he might catch a glimpse of mine. Though in these interactions the expected sound did not materialise, the boy was well aware of what might, or should, have been there and yet was not there due to his interventions.

It was here that the boy, in an ironic and conscious twist, praised our – silent – play as a great musical achievement and called the two of us 'true artists', which became a much repeated, varied and humorous part of our sessions.

However, it was noteworthy that I could observe this third phase of enhanced symbolic abilities only in the three blind children who had no added learning disability. The other three children with an added disability seemed to remain at the developmental threshold around the onset of symbolisation.

Summarising my insights from the third developmental phase, it seems that here children actively started limiting or 'clipping' our musical plays into a symbolic shape that they could increasingly control. Here, the absence of sound gained a prominent position. I suggest that in this case, an absence, that is, a silence, *consciously induced by the child,* was able to evoke a presence, that is, a sound – which the boy knew would or should be there, and yet was not.

Discussion of findings

In the following section, I will scrutinise my findings in relation to the literature and to the three research questions as they emerged from the literature review.

The first question was: In which way can music therapy be helpful for the congenitally blind child's ego development?

The study's base assumption was that the musical process in music therapy displays and changes the specific relationship between the blind child and the sighted therapist by enhancing the children's ability to symbolise. The findings show that this assumption generally held true; the children gradually learned to initiate, respond to and regulate or terminate contact; their understanding and differentiation of 'me' versus 'not-me' emerged gradually, including their understanding and awareness of their body boundaries and their body as distinct from my body. They began to address me by my first name. Eventually, the children's emerging ability to create, use and understand symbols can be regarded as the pivot of ego development. I will return to these particular concerns when looking at the third research question.

While I had assumed and confirmed the children's growing ego development from the case material, the exact nuts and bolts became much clearer when extrapolating three distinct developmental phases that seemed to govern such a development:

1. Arranging nameless forms to sequential chains and developing the expectation of a musical event to happen.
2. Forming rhythmic trajectories from acoustic fragments.
3. Developing narratives from such timed structures.

The second research question was concerned with the role that music can play in enhancing ego development, that is, what kinds of interactional forms and which kind of scenes can be observed?

The interactional forms, as they occurred in the developmental phases, showed to be:

PHASE 1: Here, I needed to initiate contact, holding the child, mirroring the child's sounds, offering sounds and describing the physical and acoustic phenomena.

PHASE 2: As I gradually withdrew from holding the child, or offering sounds, the child increasingly became the initiator of musical impulses, repetitions and cycles. The children began to utilise me to lean flexibly towards their wishes and execute their ideas.

PHASE 3: As the keyboard became the focal point of the therapeutic relationship, the children addressed me as a person and relied much less on me as someone to execute their wishes. As a new development, they played musical role-plays, commented on them and discussed them with me.

I suggest that in these scenes, music in therapy was able to provide an interactional field developing from and shifting between the sensory, the verbal and the symbolic. We can understand this with reference to Lorenzer (1970) and his ideas of the early mother–child interactions being essentially sense-based. Very similarly, the musical exchanges between my clients and myself became sensory-*symbolic* forms in phase two and even more in phase three by my reaction to them which the children picked up on and began to use themselves more actively.

The third research question asked, whether symbolisation could be observed in the investigated music therapy sessions, and if so, under which conditions?

The ability to symbolise gradually developed in the three children without a learning disability over the second and the third developmental phase. Once they had learned to anticipate a sound (that I carried into the session and into our relationship), to initiate it independently, to structure and to repeat it, they increasingly began to assign meaning to their musical activities.

This can be understood through Bion's (1962a, 1962b) notion of the symbol as a response to an expectation or preconception. The children indeed anticipated and realised sounds in the first developmental phase. The second phase can equally be related to Bion's idea of 'beta elements' (sensory percepts which are experienced as meaningless or threatening 'fragments') being changed by the mother into understandable and increasingly verbalised 'alpha elements'. Such a process could be observed when the congenitally blind children and I had realised that in our relationship, sounds could not only be 'heard' but also be talked about and be woven into a meaningful narrative content emerging between us. Sound chains, born from previous fragments, had the important role of paving the way to a musical narrative as an ordered and increasingly meaningful structure. Equally crucial was the child's recognition that 'indigestible' fragments could nonetheless be contained in a useful narrative (while the mother/therapist could still be portrayed as a failing container for the child's 'sick').

The prominent role of silence or the musical pause was a surprise to me when evaluating the material; while silence seemingly and initially came across as 'empty' or 'unrelated', it emerged as a useful and self-controlled means for the blind children to structure music and narrative.

With Susanne Langer (1992), we can understand the first sounds as merely 'presentative', that is, their phenomenological aesthetic form being distinct from verbal discourse and narrative. Thus, the blind children's first phase must be regarded as paramount to their emerging musical development as much as to their psychological one: they understood that music offered them a means to create something which I, as another person, could appreciate and respond to musically without going through the abstractions of verbal discourse.

In the second phase, the experience of rhythm and repetition paved the way towards assigning symbolic meaning to the repeated sounds; this observation is supported by Gaddini (2001), who found a similar pattern of story development in child psychoanalysis. In my investigation, narratives occurring in the second developmental phase seemed yet limited and unchanging.

However, in the third phase and for the three 'only blind' children, their musical symbols became richer and more variable alongside the symbolic meaning becoming subject to verbal exchange and description. Speaking with Susanne Langer (1992) and her distinction between presentative and discursive symbolism, this was a point where the children and I became more interested in construing an increasingly *discursive* narrative for the presentative musical phenomena generated in our joint play. The third phase also marked the pivot of ego development as the children became clearly more apt to understand, use and speak about their musical play as symbolic. They realised that sounds were part of a piece of music, with a beginning and an end, with pauses and continuations.

Having answered the three research questions, I arrived at the following conclusion:

Music therapy enhanced the ego development in the study's congenitally blind children; it facilitated their transition from the sensory to the symbolic by means of an interpersonal relationship that was primarily based on the sensory while gradually introducing the verbal and the symbolic. Such a transition can be described as their progressive mastery of developmental steps that seemed organised around the understanding of music and its forms, its sounds and its silences.

Congenitally blind children without a learning disability fared much better in the development of their symbolising abilities than their peers with an added cognitive disability. This lag in the symbolisation development of the latter three blind children can only be hypothesised: it may be intrinsic to their added disability and constitute a limit of the attainable or a hurdle which takes longer to overcome; it may indicate that the role of the verbal could be key for symbol development or for detecting it. Equally possible, this prolonged lag in symbolisation may be caused by the effect of the learning disability on the interpersonal relationship. This may indicate the need of more adapted music therapy interventions or of a more suitable research methodology still to be devised. A more defined answer to this finding was beyond the scope of my current investigation which indicates that studying the interrelations between the psychodynamics of learning disability and symbolising in music therapy constitute a useful piece of future research.

Reflections on the process of investigation and its methodology

Flick (2007) advocates that even though grounded theory supposedly encourages the researcher to approach the material without intense consultation of the literature, that reading during the process of data collection is not only advisable but also crucial for the researcher. This process of category formation was a lengthy, laborious process, often leading to dead ends. Consequently, I *did* read some of the psychoanalytic literature on congenitally blind children alongside this phase of the process, which was mainly to do with my strong need, not only as a researcher but foremost as a practitioner, to understand. Therapy work was intense; being sighted, I naturally did not feel mirrored and did not receive any resonance to my visual signals or my gaze from the children; the same applied at first to any of my musical interventions, which children were initially struggling to conceptualise and did not understand as related to our relationship or to themselves. Feeling depleted and struggling with feeling ostracised from the relationship with the children, consulting the literature was my attempt to be replenished and understand this experience. In terms of countertransference, this told a tale of how the blind children's sighted mothers might feel. However, drawing my mind maps on phenomena I had observed, that is, fragments/loose forms and chains/sequences, it became increasingly clear to me that the sudden quietness in children, their vocalising and so forth did not nicely dovetail with the literature. Rather, there were always one or several elements that did not fit. This made the literature not the explaining expert research companion I had hoped for but required further thought.

As Mayring (1993) writes, the notes that a researcher makes during the phase of data collection are vital for concept formation throughout the entire research. Keeping research journals proved a useful tool; here, I had jotted down those thoughts which were related to the case material but even more with my personal need to process; they contained an abundance of thoughts and ideas, of often of poorly understood first time impressions and my attempts to grasp what I had encountered. They were certainly a lifesaver in terms of my lack of blind-specific supervision and to contain and understand the essence of the therapeutic situation in retrospect.

Unexpected findings and areas of further research

Unsurprisingly, the sequence of developmental steps was unexpected and became, as I started formulating first ideas while still practicing, a relief and an aide for my practice. When I entered my work with the blind, I was a novice to the field and consequently struggled with our emerging relationship, the initial absence of symbolisation and the fragmented nature of the blind children's early utterances. Their blindness did not simply determine the relationship, but blindness, as such, became symbolic at times. This manifested as my feeling that something was missing, that there was a gap, which could not be exclusively assigned to the child; in other words, it was not the child who was determined by his or her sensory deficit, but the sensory gap between us, as such, created a deep feeling of isolation and mismatch. My countertransference reactions could be signified by a deep sense of uncertainty, as I did not receive any response to my gazes and my mimics.

At times I became extremely upset when, outside sessions and in my daily life, I could not see things, or when listening to classical music felt that this 'perfect' unfragmented form would, somehow, be a 'lie' – while Jazz and its fragmentations would feel more 'true'. Therefore, an enquiry into the music therapist's countertransference reactions to blindness would be another subject for investigation and shed more light onto the ramifications of the relationship between sighted music therapist and blind child.

Another area that emerged and has not been part of this current investigation was my observations and insights into the relationship between the sighted parents and their blind children. The parents' need for support and for having someone to cater to their difficulties in their emotional relationship with their children was immense. As I regularly talked to them on how music therapy developed with their children, I noticed that they seemed happy and became interested. This seemed grounded in the fact that someone else could see something in their children and would explain something about their children to them that they did not and could not. They seemed eager to absorb anything to highlight their child's individuality. Such a need reflects Fraiberg's insights from the 1970s, which led her to develop a programme for parents of blind children to enhance their interactions and understanding.

My meetings with parents could have been intensified and made more frequent and prominent, but due to the restraints of this research project in terms of time and financial resources, this proved impossible. Also, this need to foster the parents' understanding of their children and to mediate their relationships might best be catered for in a different construct, that is, with second person involved, to avoid role confusions. Investigating this parent–child relationship by using music therapy as an intervening agent might be an important piece of future research in music therapy.

References

Aepkers, F. (2008) *Mit deinen Augen. Musiktherapie mit blinden Kindern und Jugendlichen.* Saarbrücken: VDM.

Aepkers, F., and Stark, A. (2005) 'Musiktherapie in einer Schule für Blinde' in Tüpker, R. et. al. (eds.) *Musiktherapie in der Schule.* Wiesbaden: Reichert, pp. 125–136.

Bion, W.R. (1962a) *Learning from Experience.* London: Karnac.

Bion, W.R. (1962b) 'A theory of thinking', *International Journal of Psychoanalysis,* 43, pp. 306–310.

Bishop, M., Hobson, R.P., and Lee, A. (2005) 'Symbolic play in congenitally blind children', *Development in Psychopathology,* 17, pp. 447–465. https://doi.org/10.1017/S0954579405050212

Burlingham, D. (1961) Some notes on the development of the blind. *Psychoanalytic Study of the Child,* 16, pp. 121–145.

Burlingham, D. (1965) Some problems of ego-development in blind children. *Psychoanalytic Study of the Child,* 20, pp. 194–208.

Codding, P. (2000) 'Music therapy literature and clinical applications for blind and severely visually impaired persons: 1940–2000', in *Effectiveness of music therapy procedures: Documentation of research and clinical practice.* Silver Spring, MD: The American Music Therapy Association.

Flick, U. (2007) *Qualitative Sozialforschung. Eine Einführung.* Hamburg: Rowohlt Taschenbuch Verlag.

Fraiberg, S. (1968) 'Parallel and divergent patterns in blind and sighted infants', *Psychoanalytic Study of the Child,* 23, pp. 264–300.

Fraiberg, S. (1969) 'Libidinal object constancy and mental representation', *Psychoanalytic Study of the Child,* 24, pp. 9–47.

Fraiberg, S. (1971) 'Separation crisis in two blind children', *Psychoanalytic Study of the Child,* 26, pp. 355–371.

Fraiberg, S. (1977a) Congenital sensory and motor deficits and ego formation. *Annual of Psychoanalysis,* 5, pp. 169–194.

Fraiberg, S. (1977b) *Insights from the blind. Comparative studies of blind and sighted infants.* New York: Basic Books.

Fraiberg, S. (1979) 'Blind infants and their mothers: an examination of the sign system' in Bullowa, M. (ed.), *Before speech. The beginning of interpersonal communication.* Cambridge: Cambridge University Press, pp. 149–169.

Fraiberg, S., and Adelson, E. (1973) 'Self-representation in language and play: Observations of blind children', *Psychoanalytic Quarterly,* 42, pp. 539–562.

Fraiberg, S., and Freedman, D.A. (1964) 'Studies in the ego development of the congenitally child', *Psychoanalytic Study of the Child,* 19, pp. 113–169.

Fraiberg, S., Siegel, B.L., and Gibson, R. (1966) 'The role of sound in the search behavior of a blind infant', *Psychoanalytic Study of the Child*, 21, pp. 327–357.

Gaddini, E. (2001) *Das Ich ist vor allem ein körperliches. Beiträge zur Psychoanalyse der ersten Strukturen.* Tübingen: Edition Diskord.

Glaser, B.G., and Strauss, A.L. (2005) *Grounded theory. Strategien qualitativer Forschung.* Bern: Huber.

Gruber, H., and Hammer, A. (eds.) (2002) *Ich sehe anders. Medizinische, psychologische und pädagogische Grundlagen der Blindheit und Sehbehinderung bei Kindern.* Würzburg: Edition Bentheim.

Kern, P. (2006a) 'Connecting and learning through music: Music therapy for young children with visual impairments and their families', *Music Therapy Today*, VII(1), (March), 99–105. [Online]. Available at: http://www.musictherapyworld.net

Kern, P. (2006b) 'Music therapy for infants and toddlers with visual impairments', *Early Childhood Newsletter*, Vol. 12(10), June.

Langer, S. (1992) *Philosophie auf neuem Wege – Das Symbol im Denken, im Ritus und in der Kunst.* Frankfurt: Fischer.

Lorenzer, A. (1970) *Sprachzerstörung und Rekonstruktion. Vorarbeiten zu einer Metatheorie der Psychoanalyse.* Frankfurt: Suhrkamp.

Mayring, P. (1993) *Einführung in die qualitative Sozialforschung. Eine Anleitung zu qualitativem Denken.* Weinheim: Beltz Psychologie-Verlags-Union.

McLeod, J. (2003) *Doing counselling research.* London: SAGE.

Metell, M. (2015) '"A great moment … because of the music": An exploratory study on music therapy and early interaction with children with visual impairment and the sighted caregivers. *British Journal of Visual Impairment*, 33, pp. 111–125.

Orff, G. (1982) 'Der Wert des akustischen Phänomens und des prämelodischen Spiels in der Entwicklung eines blinden Mädchens', *Musiktherapeutische Umschau*, 3(4), pp. 283–293.

Stern, D.N. (1990) *Diary of a baby.* New York: Basic Books.

Warren, D.H. (1984) *Blindness and early childhood development.* New York: American Foundation for the Blind.

Wills, D.M. (1965) 'Some observations on blind nursery school children's understanding of their world', *Psychoanalytic Study of the Child*, 20, pp. 344–364.

Wills, D.M. (1968) 'Problems of play and mastery in the blind child', *British Journal of Medical Psychology*, 41, pp. 213–222.

Wills, D.M. (1979a) 'Early speech development in blind children', *Psychoanalytic Study of the Child*, 34, pp. 85–117.

Wills, D.M. (1979b) 'The ordinary devoted mother and her blind baby', *Psychoanalytic Study of the Child*, 34, pp. 31–49.

Wills, D.M. (1981) 'Some notes on the application of the diagnostic profile to young blind children', *Psychoanalytic Study of the Child*, 36, pp. 217–237.

8

DRAMA, YOUTH AND CHANGE: THE DRAMATIC SELF HYPOTHESIS AS A TOOL TO UNDERSTAND PERSONALITY DISORDERS IN ADOLESCENCE

Salvo Pitruzzella

> *The force that through the green fuse drives the flower*
> *Drives my green age; that blasts the roots of trees*
> *Is my destroyer.*
> *And I am dumb to tell the crooked rose*
> *My youth is bent by the same wintry fever.*
> (Dylan Thomas, 1933)

> *Dearest Father, what becomes of the boy*
> *No longer a boy? Please —*
> *What becomes of the shepherd*
> *When the sheep are cannibals?*
> (Ocean Vuong, 2016)

1 Adolescence and identity: a false myth?

Adolescence is said to be a time of paradoxes. It is a time when biological and mental strength are at their apex, but also a time when the rates of morbidity and mortality increase by 200%. It is a time when thinking and reasoning abilities make a leap, but in this time, the propensity for reckless and dangerous behaviour is dramatically increased (Dahl, 2004: 3).

In the 1960s, Erik Erikson sketched a powerful timeline of our individual human development. He started from the premise that 'people's innate need for a psycho-social identity is anchored to their socio-genetic evolution' (Erikson, 1968: 45). In his view, human life is composed of phases of development, which are not homogeneous; each of them is marked by a different existential conflict. The passage from one phase to another is not smooth and gradual but consists of a 'psycho-social crisis', from which one can come out with an enhanced identity, only if a new value emerges from the crisis. Adolescence is particularly marked by the conflict between a clear identity and a confused and fragmented one. Erikson's stance is perfectly placed in its time: the twentieth century has been marked by the 'identity obsession' (Remotti, 2010). It inherited the idea of nation from the previous century, and took it to its extreme consequences, while at the same time what for centuries had been at the roots of people's identities, the local cultures imbued with what Ivan Illich has called 'vernacular values', were gradually erased worldwide and substituted by the overflowing mass culture. On the other hand, the same century had started with a conspicuous searching into the depths of individual mind, which marked the birth of psychology, from the early introspection method to Freud's psychoanalysis, which can be construed as an earnest quest for a 'real' Self, our true identity. But this was long before the postmodern turn in world culture disarranged identity's very notion, turning it into what Kenneth Gergen has called 'multiphrenia', 'the splitting of the individual into a multiplicity of self-investments' (Gergen, 1991: 73), none of which plays the role of identity's spokesperson. As we are well aware, this effect has been multiplied by the new media: on the web, identities can be effortlessly invented, exposed, played and changed at will, with no relation at all with a 'core' personal identity.

Therefore, two elements should be taken into consideration when discussing therapy with adolescents.

First, we must be aware that the commonly held idea of identity is a double-edged sword. At a social and cultural level, it can be a reassuring anchor in a time of uncertainty; on the other hand, it is at the roots of the nefarious divide between 'we' and 'the others' that engender what the Lebanese-French writer Amin Malouf calls 'murderous identities' (*identités meurtrières*) (Malouf, 1998). And since therapy does not exist in a void, the social and cultural features that influence the process of growing in adolescence must be thoroughly interrogated. The prolonged exposure to a seemingly unending world crisis has enhanced young people's feelings of fear and anxiety about the future, and eventually turned them towards nihilism and depression-like passive resignation (Benasayag and Schmit, 2007; Galimberti, 2007). In this, Erikson was half right: this period of life is connoted by a compulsive search. However, it is not so much a search for identity, but rather for identification and for recognition: being part of a group and being recognised by it, either large or small, actual or virtual, seems to become a necessity for adolescents, even though the results of the identification are no more than, quoting Gergen, '*pastiche* personalities' or 'ersatz beings'.

Second, we should consider this fragmentation not as a pathology in itself, but rather as a condition with which we must come to terms. And also here Erikson was half right: adolescence is actually a 'psycho-social crisis', and as such is a time of risks and opportunities, but its main focus is not on how to frame a steady and safe identity, but on being in the flow of transformation, to avoid being submerged by it. Learning how to surf upon the waves of this flow, a surfing/selfing rather than a compact Self. Yet it is also important to take into account how mental disorders that often seem to start in this time are strictly connected with the tremendous power of this flow, but at the same time are structured by the changes occurring in the adolescent brain and mind, which we will briefly examine.

2 The adolescent brain

Our brain development during our lifetime is not a cumulative and gradual process: it goes through periods of rapid transformations, in which it is not a matter of integrating the change into a system, but of totally rearranging the whole system in order to survive the change (Benasich and Ribary, 2018). Adolescence is one of these thresholds. We should not forget that for a very long time human beings had rites of passage, where this radical transformation was celebrated by the whole community. Even though there are fewer studies on the adolescent brain, compared to adult and child studies, neurosciences have substantially confirmed the whole picture. However, there are some details in current research that are worth noting, as they offer challenging points of view on how the picture is framed.

There is evidence, based on the comparison between the human brain and other mammalian brains, that the hormonal explosion at this age triggers many different brain processes, accelerating some of them while slowing down others (Blakemore, Burnett and Dahl, 2010; Casey, Jones and Somerville, 2011).

Pruning and myelinisation are quite interesting cases. The neuronal connections in our brain grow vertiginously since birth, and the learning child's brain is literally full of active chains of neurons; this, of course, improves imagination but reduces efficacy. Therefore, a pruning process starts in late childhood, removing obsolete neural chains; it seems that this process has a peak in adolescence (Blakemore and Choudhury, 2006; Laviola and Marco, 2011), causing a reduction of the grey matter. On the other hand, the white matter grows, as the production of myelin is improved (Paus, 2010). This means that new chains of neurons will quite rapidly substitute the old ones, and a new process of Hebbian learning (cells that fire together wire together) will start; in this time, neuroplasticity has its momentum. Therefore, the adolescent brain is substantially re-founding itself, according to some other changes that are outlined by brain research.

One of the main emerging points is the different development of the brain network related to control functions (mainly based on the prefrontal cortex), and of those related to emotions (mainly based on the limbic system). While the former grows slowly and more or less linearly, the latter has an earlier maturation. The result is that 'in emotionally salient situations, the more mature limbic system will win over the prefrontal control system. In other words, when a poor decision is made in an emotional context, the adolescent may know better, but the salience of the emotional context biases his or her behaviour in the opposite direction of the optimal action' (Casey, Jones and Hare, 2008: 116–7). This means that emotional factors, like peer pressure, drive the adolescents to undertake risky behaviours, and explain why policies of risk-prevention based on information have not had an insignificant impact on the issue (Steinberg, 2007; Casey, Getz and Galvan, 2008).

Peer pressure is also related to the improvement of what has been called the 'social brain', the complex neural network that presides over a series of cognitive functions necessary to understand others and interact with them (Blakemore, 2008). Like the brain functions, we have examined so far, the development of the social brain is not linear, and in adolescence, it has both a dramatic improvement and a threatening imbalance. It seems that 'adolescence is characterised by continuing improvement in facial emotion recognition, but that the specific developmental trajectory may differ between emotions' (Burnett et al., 2011, p. 1657). This implies that adolescents become very sensitive to emotions, but mostly to specific ones, like fear, anger and disgust, and become oversensitive to the feelings of acceptation vs rejection.

In a nutshell, this has very little to do with an identity search; it seems more an urge towards a new emotional homeostasis, which cannot be found anymore in the cradle and must be searched for outside. Fear is one of the oldest and most powerful emotional systems. In evolutionary terms, it has been one of the most efficient life-saving devices that the animal brain has ever invented, and had its role in establishing the Homo Sapiens supremacy. The problem with it is that, when activated, it can rule over all the other set of emotions (Panksepp and Biven, 2012), making hazy and uncomfortable even the most secure ones. On the other hand, the need of being accepted is connected with another basic emotion in Panksepp's classification: panic/grief, which has also been an indispensable trick to enable mammals to evolve. According to Panksepp, grief is connected with abandonment and separation, and, being a survival feature in order to claim care, is quite as powerful as fear. The adolescent brain is stormed by these strong emotions, and the need for safety turns into depending on being actively accepted by the others (Cacioppo and Patrick, 2009). Such a dependency can be so strong as to conflict with reason and overcome it.

Baruch Spinoza said that passions cannot be controlled by thought, but the only way to defeat the 'sad passions' (those under the rule of *Tristitia*) is make them overshadowed by more powerful 'joyful passions' (those under the rule of *Laetitia*). It is true that many adolescents are well equipped with a safe-attachment-related emotional gear, good enough to manage these new emotional challenges, but it is also true that for many others, the risk of succumbing and making their life a desperate, extreme and unending search is high. In this sense, the 16-year-old boy who steals his mother's car drives it drunk and kills himself and another five people (it happened two days ago in my town) is the other side of the coin of the many young people I have seen in these years, diagnosed with personality disorders, whose main problem was their inability to make friends. In the former case, peer pressure towards risk has crumbled rational control, and even shared fear had become a source of excitement (Chein et al., 2011). In the latter case, a troubled emotional balance is worsened by peer rejection, the 'sheep' become 'cannibals', and their efforts for being accepted look hazy and sometimes outlandish.

In both cases, the enormous energy delivered in this life passage, 'the force that through the green fuse drives the flower', is out of control, prey to pressing urges that cannot be fulfilled. However, I believe it can also be helped to flow causing no damage, turning instead sad passions into joyous ones.

3 The arts therapies in a day centre for adolescents

The Day Centre in which I have been working for quite a few years had the purpose of serving a target that was usually left out of the care institutions. In fact, the Children's Neuropsychiatric Service treated mostly children from first infancy to pre-pubertal age, while conversely the Adult Psychiatric Service took only people from 18 years upwards. What happens if there is an insurgence of severe psychic problems during adolescence? Usually, they are firstly ignored by the family, either because they just cannot see them, or mistakes them for 'normal' manifestations of the adolescent turmoil. But when a 15 years old boy refuses to go to school and segregates himself into his room for months in the darkness, and his parents start to get worried, they have no place to go and look for a helping hand. What often happens is that the boy's troubles grow undisturbed for years, as the family's discomfort grows, until everything breaks up, and the boy, who is now of age, is taken to an Emergency Psychiatric Ward, and will eventually enter into the psychiatric tunnel, from which it is very hard to escape.

The challenging idea of the Centre was that a focussed intervention at this time in people's life, when their brain is at the height of its plasticity, could prevent them from a career as chronic mental health service users; if not of overcoming their social difficulties, by enabling them to come to terms with them, appealing to their resources and creating spaces in which they can explore their own private world, and experiment with relationships in accepting and inclusive ways.

People with the same diagnosis can be completely different one from another, especially if they are young, so we had to devise individual strategies. It was thus important to provide a vast range of interventions, through which each client's journeys could be planned. Therefore, the Centre offered many different activities, including all the four arts therapies, discussion groups, individual counselling on demand, cookery and joinery, editing a magazine, watching and discussing films, training on instrumental skills, like using money, taking a bus, paying a bill and so on. There was also psychological support for the families, and collaboration with the schools and other educational institutions attended by the clients.

The complexity of the project was mirrored by the various approaches coexisting in the centre staff, each of them presenting a different paradigm for understanding reasons and suggesting remedies. Putting together all the points of view was not an easy task: we spent a lot of time discussing any single case, comparing the diverse interpretations and trying to find a common strategy.

However, it was commonly agreed that the arts therapies played a crucial role in the therapeutic project of the Centre, for three main reasons.

First, because they deal with emotions in a safe and manageable way. In the protected setting of the arts therapies, emotions can be expressed metaphorically and symbolically, allowing the right distance to contain them: in terms of the neuroscientific researches quoted earlier in the chapter, rebalancing the disconnected circuits presiding emotions and control.

Second, because they deal with creativity. A creative approach to life helps people to experiment with possibilities, to avoid getting stuck in dead ends and vicious circles. Practising creative arts is not just expressing one's own world through aesthetic means, but also sharing it with the others, and rearranging it accordingly.

Thirdly, because they deal with relationships. Arts therapies establish safe spaces where healthy relationships can be cultivated, which become corrective experiences that may renew people's interpersonal abilities.

In the next two sections, I will discuss in detail the specific approach of dramatherapy, and how it is connected with the themes explored so far.

4 The dramatic self hypothesis

The Dramatic Self Hypothesis is a model of human development based on a re-vision of the dramatic metaphor under the light of the deconstruction of the concept of Self mentioned earlier[1] (see Figure 8.1). I have identified NARRATIVES, ROLES, RELATIONSHIPS, and KNOWLEDGE as the *Dramatic Universals,* the essential elements through which the *dramatic reality* of the stage manifests itself, both in theatre and in dramatherapy. At the same time, they are the functions that describe how we interface with the world, what I call our *Dramatic Interface System,*

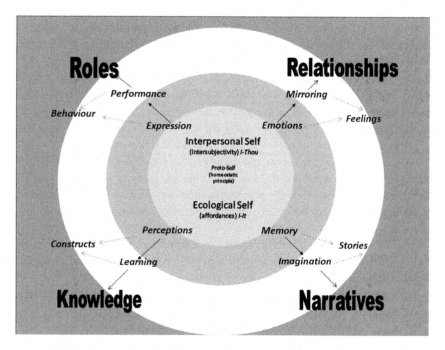

FIGURE 8.1 The dramatic self model

or *Dramatic Self*. According to the model, there is nothing like a 'core Self'; the Self is a feeling that comes out as an emergent property in a particular configuration of conscious and unconscious elements at a certain time.

Narratives are the stories we tell ourselves about ourselves and about the world, as well as the stories we tell other people about ourselves, about our version of the world, and our version of them. They can be fictional, intendedly or unwittingly. They can be told in different ways in different moments, with significant shifts in meaning. We can either strongly believe in them or just accept them suspiciously: whatever they might be, narratives shape our Self feeling.

Roles are meaningful and recognisable patterns of behaviour, through which we manifest ourselves in interpersonal situations. We are able to take and play many of them, and sometimes more than one at once. Our role repertoire affects our Self feeling.

Relationships are the fundamental result of the long evolutionary process that made us social beings. They are based on feelings and modelled by them, either being very intimate or quite shallow; they can engage us totally or just tangentially; they can be satisfactory or conflictual; they can last a whole life or just a few minutes; they can leave a deep mark in our life or remain just as faded memories: in any case, we cannot live without at least a few of them, and our experienced relationships play a crucial part in our Self feeling.

Knowledge is the sum of the constructs through which we interpret the world and anticipate the events. They are made by what we have learnt about how the world works, by experience or by instruction, and we presume could be a guide to our behaviour. Whatever its extent and coherence might be, the world version resulting from this process becomes a fundamental piece of our Self feeling.

Our narratives, roles, relationships, and knowledge can be partly under the light of consciousness, but the processes producing them are partially unconscious; this is why they cannot be easily changed by our conscious efforts. They are interdependent from each other, but each of them is developed along separate lines that begin from the basic features through which newborn babies encounter the world.

They are rooted in biological endowments: the emotion-expression system is the tool evolution invented to help newborn human mammals to establish bonds with their conspecifics, while the perception-memory system is there to help them in dealing with their environment. They do not need consciousness to work, and they will keep working for most of our lives. However, these biological functions are modified by our encounters with others and with the material and cultural world we are immersed in. In other words, we entertain with others and with the world an intersubjective and enactive relationship (Pitruzzella, 2016).

As experience expands, the feeling of a conscious self emerges gradually in a timespan that ranges from first infancy to adolescence.

Memory provides the materials upon which Imagination can exert its power. Imagination rearranges, recombines and transforms maps and images that are generated by perceptual elements, either conscious or not, and fills the gaps of Memory. At an enhanced consciousness level, the Memory/Imagination process produces conscious Stories.

Expressions, through the continuous feedback from other people, as well as through our mimetic tendency, become Performances, in which intentionality and direction of the expression are clear, as well as are our expectations of the responses to them. Children become so clever in performing that they use this skill for make-believe play, but they also learn to perform fake expressions, intended to influence others. At an enhanced consciousness level, the Expression/Performance process produces conscious Behaviour.

'Emotions' activate the process of 'Mirroring' and are modified by it. We know that perceiving another's emotions triggers our mirror systems, producing an embodied simulation of that emotion. The first emotional exchanges between infant and caregiver have set this process in motion; as the baby grows, mirrors multiply, and this enlarged experience helps them to fine-tune their emotional processes according to the social environment. They develop emotional tools to understand others and the interpersonal frames. At an enhanced consciousness level, the Emotions/Mirroring process produces what we experience as conscious Feelings.

Perceptions are the bases for Learning: all we learn, either by experience, by imitation or by instruction, goes through our perceptive organs. What children learn feeds back on their perceptive systems, modifying their functioning accordingly. Learning influences their system of expectations, that is how they interpret new perceptive inputs according to their previous maps. At an enhanced consciousness level, the Perception/Learning process produces conscious Constructs.

Stories, behaviours, feelings and constructs and the raw materials through which our conscious self is formed as an emerging property of the continuous rearrangements of the whole system in time. Adolescence is the most momentous of all these re-arrangements; it is the time when they start manifesting themselves as NARRATIVES, ROLES, RELATIONSHIPS and KNOWLEDGE. If we read it in the light of the earlier discussed research, it seems that the process of brain re-foundation triggered by the pruning/myelinisation process that is in motion in adolescence is crucial in the production of the conscious Self. And we can see how difficult it can be at a time when your emotional side is overwhelming.

The idea of dramatherapy is that playing freely with these elements in a special space, safe and emotionally warm may trigger processes of reworking and rearranging them, which can be addressed towards a healthy balance between thought and emotions. In this sense, the dramatic process is a light and aware recapitulation of the painstaking making of the individual self. Therefore, in its status of a miniature world within which all sort of experiments can be made, it gives permission to be creative.

5 The adolescent drama

M. is a girl attending the Centre whose diagnosis is 'schizotypal personality disorder'. She is 17, but she looks much younger, being leaner and shorter than her peers, and wears heavy prescription glasses. When she was adopted at age of five, she presented evident signs of malnutrition. She manifests a certain childish awkwardness, coupled with a remarkable intelligence and memory. Familiar care helped her to live a quite serene childhood, and the family had proved good enough to balance the affects when a new unexpected baby arrived when M. was ten. M.'s poor physical conditions have been compensated by her vivid intelligence. She had first grades at the primary school, and tolerated the change to the secondary, even though she had to leave her few childhood friends and had some difficulties with new acquaintances. In the first year of high school, she was victim of a series of bullying episodes, which triggered a profound crisis. She started having eating disorders and recurrent nightmares that bordered on somnambulism. She decided to drop out of school, and when her parents tried to challenge her, had explosive tantrums that brought her to the threshold of epilepsy-like attacks. For a long year, she had lived segregated in her room, until eventually her parents convinced her to go for help. Actually, she did not regret her year of 'exile': she was never bored, she saw a lot of movies, especially cartoons, read history books and studied Wikipedia, to the point that she had learnt by heart quite a lot of entries. She said she was here as a favour she was doing for her parents.

When she first came to the dramatherapy group, I asked her to turn off her phone before entering the room, which she dutifully did (actually, I never saw her using it, except for calling her parents at the end of the day). However, she insisted in keeping the phone pendant which had a stuffed bear attached to it that was larger than the phone itself. When I asked her if she preferred to put it aside, she retorted that she felt authorised to keep it because the rules on personal belongings referred only to phones. I could not reply to such a well-conceived argument, so she kept the bear, using it at the beginning as a sort of middle way between a transitional object and an amulet to protect her against the challenging new group of people she had just entered. The group had already been formed for about six months (three boys and two girls), it was closely knit and had found its own way of working. I would say, its own *poetics*, which, if I may, reminds me some characteristics of the glorious post-war Italian cinema (first of all the great Vittorio De Sica), swinging from social tragedy to romantic comedy: the preferred scenes were of violent crimes or of embarrassing love intrigues. When asked to join some improvisation, she often declined by pushing the bear forward, as a sign of refusal. Gradually, the friendly atmosphere of the group started soothing her diffidence, and she began to try and play some minor characters in the stories proposed by the others. In these cases, she left the bear on the chair and tried, in her way, to cope.

In a scene where she acted an old lady victim of a bag-snatcher, instead of falling down as it was expected, she kept her bag steady and reacted to the aggressor in a rather assertive way. A., the other actor, protested: 'In *real life* you cannot do it! In *real life* you just bloody well fall and cry!' 'Yes, but I was a kung-fu black belt!' A., with an Indiana Jones-like move, extracts a gun and fires. M. feigns to be shot, sets up a melodramatic pantomime, with horrible sights and shouts, and finally collapses on the floor, whispering: 'I am dying ... You vile assassin ... Oh, revenge me, I plead!', getting a big applause from the audience. With some mumbling, A. goes along with it, and since then, they became good partners in any kind of improvisation. Yes, because the genres of the improvisations were going soon to be updated.

The more M. sensed herself to be accepted by the group, the more she used her wit and her talent in the service of the others, providing clever suggestions that raised the level of the performance, and, consequently, the group's enjoyment. And the more she joyously played with the group, the more fear was losing its grip upon her. Eventually, she felt free to propose her favourite scenarios, which were mostly based on fantasy or 'magic realism' (like some ghost stories), and switched the group poetics from 'naturalism' to 'symbolism'. She convinced the group to play her stories, although they were complex and philosophical, and sometimes too entangled to be understood properly (especially by the boys, who were more inclined to action). Gradually, she started asking to play some key roles in the stories, usually as a heroine, a wise princess or a good witch, using often her toy bear as a sceptre or as a magic wand. The other members of the group complied with it: it was not the first time that a member of the group claimed his or her space, and became for a while the protagonist, not only of the stories staged, but also of the group passionate care. This did not prevent some 'old style' stories from being proposed from time to time, but it was clear that now was M.'s time, and she should be supported in using the dramatic space to explore whatever she wished to explore. The period of about two months when M. played as a protagonist coincided with a visible change in her behaviour in the other moments in the Centre: she was more sociable in the leisure time, and refrained from using her prodigious memory to humiliate the adversaries in board games; she started accepting uncomplainingly the counselling sessions (which she had loathed so far); collaborated in the cooking group; and lastly, she became friends with one of the other girls, and invited her home to watch a movie together.

The dramatic process, like all complex processes, it is not a progressive and cumulative one, but it is rather punctuated by special moments which mark discontinuities and qualitative leaps. These special moments are often turning points in the journey undertaken by both the individual and the group within the *dramatic reality*. During these moments, it almost seems that a multitude of fragments scattered along the way in the previous dramatic work suddenly take on visible form, often in the shape of symbolic structures. In a quite old article in the *Dramatherapy Journal*, I called these moments *States of Grace*: 'after these events, people show undeniable signs that 'something has changed'. They are more relaxed, more open to communication and relationship; they seem to enjoy more the things they do. Often these signs are also visible in the 'external world', in people's everyday life, and they foreshadow further lasting transformations. Almost always they are visible thresholds in the growth of people's dramatic abilities. This opens us to the possibility that the dramatic process can reach further healing steps' (Pitruzzella, 2002). The 'old lady' scene had been a *State of Grace* in M.'s progress; the 'rescue of the slaves' was another one, her last 'crucial scene' in the dramatherapy group.

One day she enters the dramatherapy room which a strange smirk on her face, saying she has a new story to play which includes a surprise. It is the story of a drought-stricken African tribe, which sends a group of explorers to look for new springs. She will take the role of Amallah, the shaman woman, owner of a magic talisman (her bear), which has the virtues of finding water and protecting against enemies. They come across a hidden spring quite soon, but they are attacked by a gang of slave-hunters, attempting to catch them. M. tells the story up to this point and then the improvisation starts. True surprise comes soon after, as, in the middle of the ambush, Amallah declares to her companions that the talisman suddenly has ceased to work; they are captured by the slavers and put in chains. From now on, she ceases being the leader of the play, and the decision about what to do is passed on to the group. After a first moment of bafflement, they simply choose to fight their way through (which is quite different from the abstruse plot M. could have devised). After a stylised and exhilarating fake-fight (in which my assistant and I played the slavers), the explorers come back to their village, and celebrate their victory with a joyous dance with drums and bells, involving the whole group. At the end, I privately asked M. if she would need the bear anymore, and she answered: 'No. But I will keep it as a souvenir.

This was M.'s goodbye and swan song. In the following months, she was discharged from the Centre. After that, she went back to school and resumed some of her friendships. As far as I know, she is now studying history at University and has a fiancé. As the resources of the Centre were manifold, it is not easy to tell whether dramatherapy has been cause of her change or just witness of it. In her year in the group, she had been playing roles, inventing narratives, establishing relationships and attuning her knowledge system. And all this could happen in safe, non-judging environment, where 'sheep' are not 'cannibals', and people take care of each other. In this space, emotions can be handled through the magic of dramatic reality, and everyday reality can be transformed by the shared experience of creating.

Conclusion

As the resources of the Centre were manifold, it is not easy to tell whether dramatherapy has been cause of her change or just witness of it. What I can notice is that her progress in the group can be easily explained according to our model. As we hinted earlier, the *Dramatic Interface System* can get stuck: roles can become masks to protect and conceal ourselves; relationships tangled traps in which we toil to survive; narratives and knowledge stagnant descriptions of an inexorably gloomy reality. The *Dramatic Self* loses its flexibility, and, instead of being a resource to cope with the always changing flow of life, turns into a burden that hinders the possibility of a creative engagement with the world. In her time in the dramatherapy group, M's rigid defensive trenches had not been directly attacked: her Hermione-Granger-like *Persona*, intelligent, childish and self-conscious, had been welcomed and accepted at face value, so was her awkward and suspicious way of endeavouring relationships. Neither her narratives about herself nor her peculiar worldview had been challenged. This non-judging attitude, which has been cultivated until it became the group's Golden Rule, and the affective warmth and emotional containment it entails were already there when M. entered the group. They gradually melted the stronghold into which she had turned the elements of her *Dramatic Self*. In the safe and free space of the *dramatic reality*, she could allow these rigid features to be loosened a bit, and she could experiment with new roles, inventing new narratives, attempting new ways to establishing relationships and attuning her knowledge system with the others. Did this whole process of change affect the basic levels of the emotion-expression and the memory-perception system, and accordingly trigger a rebalancing process at the brain level? This cannot be proved but can be hoped for. All we can say is that M. seemed to succeed in allowing her *joyful passions* to overcome her *sad passions*. And at the very end, with her *state of grace*, she showed us how a new story can be a sign and a symbol of change. All this could happen in a place where 'sheep' are not 'cannibal', and people take care of each other – a space where emotions can be handled through the magic of dramatic reality, and everyday reality can be transformed by the shared experience of creating.

I believe that dramatherapy, being based on the multiform art of theatre, is flexible enough to cope with the complexity of mental health disorders in adolescence, which combines the unpredictability of the brain with some unescapable psycho-social bonds. Unpredictability may open the doors to creativity, and the urges triggered by the social brain can be soothed by group empathy. Through drama, the wonderful potentiality of the adolescent mind can be used to explore their narratives, roles, relationships and knowledge, enhancing their power over their emotions through rediscovering joy and care.

Note

1 I had first presented this model at the ECArTE Conference 2019, in Alcalà De Henares (Spain), in a long paper from which some of the materials of this chapter are taken. The unabridged version of the text will be published in the forthcoming ECArTE book (2021). An expanded version of the model is going to be the main topic of my next book.

References

Benasayag, M., and Schmit, G. (2007) *Les passions tristes. Souffrance psychique et crise sociale.* Paris: Editions La Découverte.

Benasich, A., and Ribary, U. (2018) *Emergent brain dynamics. Prebirth to adolescence.* Cambridge: MIT Press.

Blakemore, S.J. (2008) 'The social brain in adolescence', *Nature Reviews Neuroscience,* 9(4), pp. 267–277.

Blakemore, S.-J., Burnett, S., and Dahl, R.E. (2010) 'The role of puberty in the developing adolescent brain', *Human Brain Mapping,* 31(6), pp. 926–933.

Blakemore, S.-J., and Choudhury, S. (2006) 'Development of the adolescent brain: implications for executive function and social cognition', *Journal of Child Psychology & Psychiatry,* 47(3/4), pp. 296–312.

Burnett, S., Sebastian, C., Cohen Kadosh, K., and Blakemore, S.-J. (2011) 'The social brain in adolescence', *Neuroscience & Biobehavioral Reviews,* 35(8), pp. 1654–1664.

Cacioppo, J.T., and Patrick, W. (2009) *Loneliness. Human nature and the need for social connection.* New York: Norton.

Casey, B.J., Getz, S., and Galvan, A. (2008). 'The adolescent brain', *Developmental Review,* 28, pp. 62–77.

Casey, B.J., Jones, R.M., and Hare, T.A. (2008) 'The adolescent brain', *Annals of the New York Academy of Sciences,* 1124, pp. 111–126.

Casey, B.J., Jones, R.M., and Somerville, L.H. (2011) 'Braking and accelerating of the adolescent brain', *Journal of Research on Adolescence,* 21(1), pp. 21–33.

Chein, J., Albert, D., O'Brien, L., Uckert, K., and Steinberg, L. (2011) 'Peers increase adolescent risk taking by enhancing activity in the brain's reward circuitry', *Developmental Science,* 14(2), pp. F1–F10.

Dahl, R.E. (2004) 'Adolescent brain development – a period of vulnerabilities and opportunities', *Annals of the New York Academy of Sciences,* 1021, pp. 1–22.

Erikson, E.H. (1968). *Identity. Youth and crisis.* New York: Norton & Company.

Galimberti, U. (2007). *L'ospite inquietante. Il nichilismo e i giovani.* Milano: Feltrinelli.

Gergen, K. (1991). *The saturated self.* New York: Basic Books.

Laviola, G., and Marco, E.M. (2011) 'Passing the knife edge in adolescence- Brain pruning and specification of individual lines of development', *Neuroscience & Biobehavioral Reviews,* 35(8), pp. 1631–1633.

Malouf, A. (1998) *Les identités meurtrières.* Paris: Grasset.

Paus, T. (2010) 'Growth of white matter in the adolescent brain: Myelin or Axon?' *Brain Cognition,* 72(1), pp. 26–35.

Panksepp, J., and Biven, L. (2012) *The archaeology of mind: Neuroevolutionary origins of human emotions.* New York: Norton.

Pfeifer, J.H., and Allen, N.B. (2012) 'Arrested development. Reconsidering dual-systems models of brain function in adolescence and disorders', *Trends in Cognitive Sciences,* 16(6), pp. 322–329.

Pitruzzella, S. (2002) 'States of grace. Transformative events in dramatherapy', *Dramatherapy Journal,* 24(2), pp. 3–9.

Pitruzzella, S. (2016) *Drama, creativity and intersubjectivity: Roots of change in dramatherapy.* London: Routledge.

Remotti, F. (2010) *L'ossessione identitaria.* Bari: Laterza.

Steinberg, L. (2007) 'Risk taking in adolescence: new perspectives from brain and behavioral science', *Current Directions in Psychological Science,* 16(2), pp. 55–59.

Steinberg, L. (2015) *Age of opportunity. Lessons from the new science of adolescence.* New York: Mariner Books.

Thomas, D. (1933). The force that through the green fuse drives the flower', *The collected poems of Dylan Thomas: The centenary edition (2016).* John Goodby, UK: Weidenfeld & Nicolson, p. 43.

Thomas, D. (2014) *The collected poems of Dylan Thomas: The centenary edition.* London: Weidenfeld & Nicolson.

Vuong, O. (2016) *Night sky with exit wounds.* Port Townsend, WA: Copper Canyon Press.

9

AN ART THERAPY CLINIC FOR CHILDREN WITH HEART CONDITIONS: TOWARDS INTERDISCIPLINARY RESEARCH OF AN INNOVATIVE SERVICE

Sheena McGregor, Karen McLeod, and Michael Morton

Introduction

This chapter describes an innovative art therapy practice for children diagnosed with chronic heart conditions and focuses on children who display symptoms of distress, anxiety and anger, but are unable to engage with talking therapies. The authors describe the experience from the perspective of three different disciplines, art therapy (Sheena McGregor), cardiology (Dr Karen McLeod), and liaison psychiatry (Dr Michael Morton), who were concerned with the distress found in this group of children, and collaborated closely to establish an art therapy service to support the children's adaptation to their illness. The presentation of two case studies illustrates the development of the service. The first case was instrumental in the development of the approach and eventually led to establishing a Cardiac Art Therapy Clinic, and the second case set within the already fully functioning service catering to larger numbers of children with chronic heart disease. This is followed by the reflections of the art therapist, consultant paediatric cardiologist, consultant paediatric liaison psychiatrist, children and children's parents on the development of this approach, from its instigation based on a single case to the subsequent development of a specialised service. These thoughts are accompanied by brief, exemplary verbatim comments on art therapy from children's parents and a child, and a section on the crucial role of the cardiac nurses as co-therapists. The Paediatric Liaison Psychiatry Consultant's contribution further details service development and focuses on children's needs and art therapy's role in their treatment. Feedback is presented from a structured interview the Consultant Paediatric Cardiologist. The discussion will present perspectives, outline key practice issues and pinpoint questions and objectives for future research. The chapter scrutinises how the children's psychological needs are entwined with their physical ones, calling for a new, expert and interdisciplinary art therapy service, which, in turn, has stimulated research interest.

The art therapist's perspective

As a trainee art therapist, my final placement was in a child psychiatric in-patient setting where I ran a weekly art therapy group with nursing support. The team was headed by a consultant child psychiatrist, Dr Michael Morton, my co-author, whose only stipulation was that all children should attend. Staff interest in the images created by the children encouraged me to take the artwork to the weekly multi-disciplinary team meeting. In one instance, I brought clay containers made by a child with an early onset eating disorder, as these spoke so eloquently of her struggles to function as a container on any physical, emotional or psychological level (Dalley, 2006). As Miller(2016) points out, sharing is 'part of our role as arts therapists in multidisciplinary settings' in which confidentiality extends to the multiple professionals involved in the client's care (p. 23).

Some years later, I was employed in a family centre where the majority of the children referred to art therapy were in the process of being fostered or adopted following their removal from their family of origin due to extreme neglect or physical, emotional and sexual abuse. However, some referrals were made by the Family Disability Team, a specialised team within the wider Children and Families Social Work Department. The following case study concerns a child, referred to here by the pseudonym Mandy, and her mother Sally. This short case study is an abbreviated version of Mandy's long engagement with art therapy, attending 162 weekly sessions over five years.

Case Study

I was informed at the point of referral that Mandy was 11 years old and had a life expectancy in months rather than years. My first reaction was anxiety; would I be able to be with a dying child in any helpful way and not be overcome by my own feelings? I was reminded of Bion who wrote about the anxiety with which analysts can react when faced with the unknown, 'In every consulting room there ought to be two rather frightened people: the patient and the psychoanalyst. If they are not, one wonders why they are bothering to find what everyone knows' (Bion, 1990: p. 5).

Beginnings

In our first meeting, Mandy told me that she could not talk to her parents about her heart condition as they would start to cry. I realised that Mandy was used to pro-tecting adults from the pain of her life-shortening condition. She added that this was why she needed art therapy, which she was familiar with from another clinic, as she needed somewhere to bring these feelings and find a way to express them. Malchiodi (1999) suggests that art expression is particularly effective in cultivating psychological resilience in children facing chronic illness. At the start of therapy, Mandy was too unwell to attend school and was constantly with her mother. She used a wheelchair and carried an oxygen cylinder and mask at all times.

Her mother Sally stayed for part of our early sessions until she felt she could trust me with her daughter. She then waited in her car, parked outside, ready to be contacted by mobile phone if she was needed, week after week, for five years.

In a recent interview, Sally spoke about how the art therapy room, 'had everything in it'. Her reason to contribute to this paper was so that 'other mothers could have what I had'. I understand this to mean the emotional support through art therapy for Mandy, and the subsequent reduction in anxiety for the whole family. This especially applied to Sally, who needed support to confront her fears after her child being discharged from the children's hospital with her condition described as inoperable, and hopeless. Malchiodi (1999) describes a child's illness as pervading the whole family system. This was later corroborated by cardiac nurses who knew Mandy. Emotionally Mandy was robust; she rarely missed a session, showing her commitment to attending.

The commitment of her family ensured that she could attend and it functioned as a team around her. Family members occasionally took part in art therapy sessions at Mandy's invitation, and had faith in art therapy, willing to do whatever it took to support this much-loved child. I had little contact with other professionals apart from occasional meetings with the Family Disability Team. Mostly the sessions were just Mandy and me, although later, she and her mother agreed to be interviewed as participants in the writing of this chapter and were very willing to offer their perspective.

In the first session, Mandy may have been unsure how to begin but appeared in control. She said that she wanted to make a clay butterfly, and that we should both make one. In this way, she could follow my way of working without asking for help, defended against the vulnerability of not knowing how to begin. It determined our way of working together. The clay butterflies were decorated with jewels and painted in shimmering colours (Figure 9.1a and 9.1b).

Following the session, I found myself thinking how a clay butterfly is a paradox as there is no possibility of flight and butterflies represent a short but intense life. In the next session, Mandy made an image of a large, dark wing by slapping her hands covered in black paint onto a sheet of paper. Malchiodi (1999) noticed the prevalence of black in images by children with serious illness. Mandy made a large black bat from painted cardboard which she hung inside the store cupboard. This gave me a shock each time I opened the door, which I came to understand as a countertransference in relation to the fears Mandy faced on a daily basis: fears of the dark, of flying, of lifts and, most of all, of needles. Mandy also used clay to express anger. She threw lumps of clay at the walls and windows. She was encouraged to find words to identify the cause of her anger and share these with the therapist. Her anger was always a response to feeling depersonalised in health and education settings (Menzies Lyth 1988) and to not being seen as a person. Menzies Lyth 1988 Artwork as support in illness has gained growing recognition (Bach, 1966; Furth, 1988; Malchiodi, 1999; Appleton, 1993; Malchiodi, 1999; Bissonnet, 2015; Fischer, 2015; Simpson, 2015).

(a)
(b)

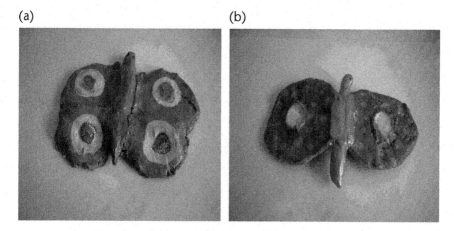

FIGURE 9.1 Clay butterflies: Clay, plastic jewels and pearlescent paint

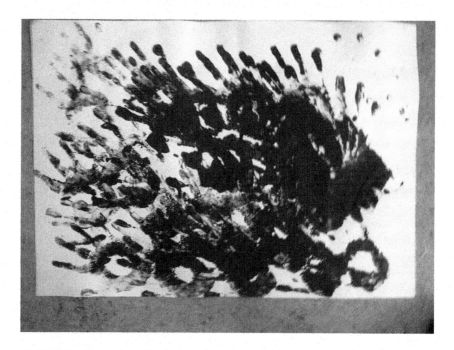

FIGURE 9.2 Dark wing: Black water-based paint, A1 paper

To help Mandy paint, I obtained a table easel and a table under which her wheelchair could fit. The more disabled Mandy was the less help she would accept. In a later interview, she spoke about her need to feel in control in art therapy, as the only area of her life this was possible; her mother waited in the car park, in case Mandy should collapse. As advised by Sally, I kept a close eye on Mandy's top lip, which would acquire a bluish tinge when she was short of oxygen (Figure 9.2).

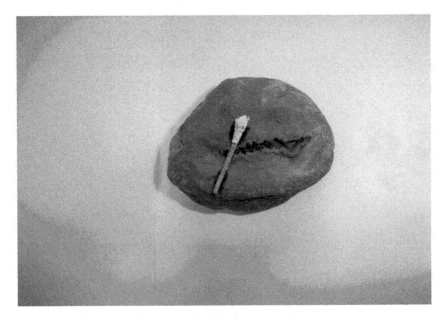

FIGURE 9.3 The stitched heart: Clay and matchstick

Work

After several months, Mandy moved away to a small table and worked with clay, with her back to me, in silence. This separation showed the capacity to be alone in the presence of another (Winnicott 1958). She then showed me a small clay heart with an incision, and a matchstick laid across the wound (Figure 9.4). She explained that this represented the operation on her heart, the matchstick being the stitch to repair the heart. In a later interview, Mandy remembered how this symbolised her taking on the role of the doctor, mending her own heart.

There followed a series of clay plaques, archaic in their essence, showing her organs with the damaged valve between the heart and lungs. It was around this time that she managed to give blood; conquering her fear of needles gave Mandy a huge sense of achievement.

As time passed, Mandy's three dimensional work included puppets made from polystyrene balls on sticks set in a clay base, their robes made from muslin soaked in paint and plaster, with hair rendered in painted cotton wool, representing the Royal Family (Figure 9.5). Her approach was messy, allowing her freedom to release the internal chaos through the expressive art processes, but always with a focused artwork as a result, elsewhere described as 'the harnessed mess', to convey the interplay between chaos and control evident in art (Birtchnell, 1984, p. 32). I was the Third Hand described by Edith Kramer, containing and supportive, but subject to her needs and direction. 'The mastery of skills or discovery of truth affords a sense of the miraculous' (Kramer, 2000, p. 49).

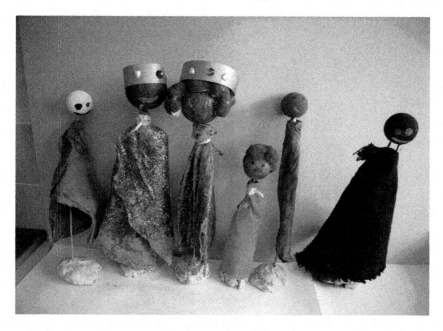

FIGURE 9.4 The Royal Family puppets: Mixed media, clay, polystyrene, fabric, cotton wool, paint and wood

Mandy worked on these over a period of years, often repainting and re-pairing the puppets which included a dark figure, a death figure who threatened the family. She was clear in her instructions that he must be kept apart when they were stored in the cupboard. Repair was often a response to anxiety around hospital appointments. The artwork reminded me of the painting 'Premonition', by John Bellany, which shows a young couple full of vigour and sensuality, surrounded by the good things of life, food, music and beauty. But, like Mandy's puppets, there is a dark figure in the background, and a ship crossing the bay outside their window, reminiscent of the boat crossing the River Styx, carrying the dead to the underworld. In my understanding, both Bellany and Mandy had the courage to acknowledge and accept the presence of death in life, which made it possible to 'live life in an authentic fashion', embracing what Heidegger (1962) called 'the state of mindfulness of being', the 'ontological mode of being in whichone can grasp the power to change oneself' (Yalom, 1980, p. 31) (see Figure 9.6).

From three dimensional pieces, Mandy went on to create a series of images using elemental materials, sand, water, flame and breath. Small circles of co-loured tissue were burnt around their edges, and the charred fragments of da-maged tissue fixed in a thick layer of glue. She gave this image the title 'Burnt Flowers', suggesting the fragility of early blossom, embodying the poignancy spoken of by Yalom. This period of work moved towards the performative as

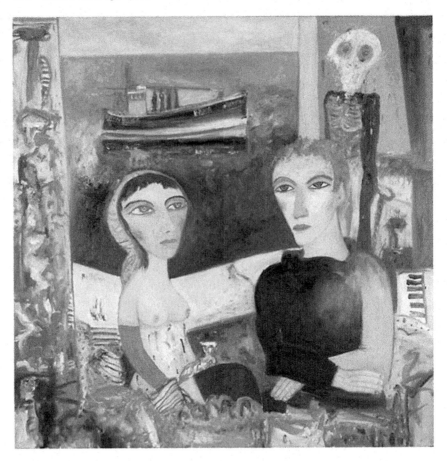

FIGURE 9.5 'Premonition', by John Bellany, 2005 (oil on canvas 60 × 60)
Source: Reproduced with the kind permission of The Estate of John Bellany, Flowers Gallery, London.

Mandy worked in a sand tray, lighting matches and candles, with water close at hand. Flames from tea lights were lit and extinguished; the symbolism was clear. Her mother could not bear to watch, as her daughter extinguished the flames over and over again. Mandy then discovered that by removing the small metal disc on the base of a tea light and floating it on water, the water would travel up the wick and extinguish the flame. The art therapist was the silent witness, the containing presence that made bearable this performance representing the extinguished flame. Shortly after this session, Mandy announced that she wanted to make a life-size model of Bruno, the family dog. She worked on this over several weeks using papier mâché, plaster and paint. Much later, in an interview, this was one of the art works she remembered.

The adventure of life and ending therapy

At school, Mandy was supervised by two classroom assistants at all times. Other children would not approach her. She was isolated and lonely until her mother intervened, and classroom assistants were asked to observe from a distance. Given space, Mandy began to make friends, in and out of school. She was now going out to play with her younger sister and friends, and made a large drawing of a real-life adventure, showing the obstacles the children had to overcome, the brambles, the rusty gate, the pipe under the bridge, the warning signs, the mud and the river. She had rescued younger children and told me that she was the bravest. Mandy attended art therapy for almost six years when she began to miss sessions, due to exams, and preparation to move on to attend college. We agreed to end therapy. On her 18th birthday, she sent me a text message, with a photograph of her dressed up to go out and celebrate with a group of friends. By the time our work drew to a close her heart appeared to have recovered enough for her to have a life and a future.

The following section describes how working with Mandy led to developing a specialised service for children with heart conditions, where they and their parents can, as Mandy's mother put it, 'have what she had'. I will revisit and scrutinise what I learned from working with Mandy and other clients when discussing the material and its potential for research.

At around the same time I began working with Mandy I was asked to run a weekly art therapy group in the child psychiatric in-patient ward of the local children's hospital. Children admitted to this ward come from all over Scotland and suffer from early onset complex mental health problems. Art therapy was seen as an integral, essential part of the treatment and developed from group provision to an approach which combined the weekly art psychotherapy group with concurrent individual sessions for all children. I was the art therapist in both modalities. The added containment (Bion, 1964; Killick, 2000; Ogden, 2004) provided by the individual sessions radically reduced acting out through aggression towards group members and staff. The children quickly understood that more private issues could be addressed in individual sessions, which allowed the group to focus on psycho-social, relational concerns, explored through interactive creative processes. As trust in the group developed, the children gradually brought the more sensitive material from individual to group sessions. Visual images were taken to team meetings and viewed as providing valuable insight into the emotional state of the children, most of whom struggled with verbalising their distress. This mentalisation approach was the basis for developing the new Cardiology Art Therapy Clinic. The role of images in assisting mentalisation (Franks and Whitaker, 2007 was understood by the team as creating a bridge between the children's inner and outer worlds, at the 'the visionary core of the therapeutic situation' (La Nave, 2015, p. 153).

Mandy's Paediatric Cardiac Consultant was aware of her long engagement with art therapy, and in discussion with Michael Morton, Paediatric Liaison Psychiatry Consultant, wondered if art therapy could help other children with heart

TABLE 9.1 Protocol for cardiac art therapy clinic

Art therapy offered in 1:1 and small group sessions

Children referred by cardiology consultants and their teams

Groups will meet fortnightly in blocks of ten sessions, with two groups running alternate weeks

Groups to meet on Fridays 3–4.15 pm with 1:1 sessions between 12.30 and 15.00 pm

Senior cardiac nurses to be co-therapists in the art therapy groups. Notes kept of all sessions, with contributions from all staff present. Regular reports to referring team.

Art work stored for duration of therapy. Images photographed and stored on Liaison Psychiatry computer.

Parents/carers to bring children to the art therapy clinic and remain in the hospital for duration of sessions.

---

conditions. Initially funded by the hospital charity for two years, this project is now in its sixth year. Over fifty children have taken part in both individual and group art therapy. Michael's interest in the images allowed these to be central to supervision.

Mandy's long engagement with art therapy had shown me that working with symbols and creative processes in a child-led approach was likely to be the most effective way of engaging children with heart conditions. Mentalisation which involves mutual reflection and creation of shared states of feeling was an aim of therapy (Shore, 2013). Interpretation was cautious as I felt it was potentially too overwhelming with such highly anxious children. The visual image contained the unspeakable (Tjasink, 2010). An important lesson I learned from working with Mandy was the need to offer art therapy in a group setting to address the social isolation and loneliness of children with heart conditions (Table 9.1).

The Pilot Project conducted in the Cardiac Art Therapy Clinic was unique in Scotland. Children attended from a wide geographical area, some travelling long distances. With very few exceptions, parents of children referred made great efforts to support regular attendance as they recognised the need for children to have contact with their peers. Informal support groups formed among the parents, meeting while their children attended art therapy.

These statements from two parents and one child stand for many others and convey their perception of the service (Box 9.1).

BOX 9.1 COMMENTS FROM PARENTS

Parent of ten-year-old boy referred with acute anxiety and fearfulness

"He was 'scared' of this (art therapy) as well – being in the hospital where he comes for treatment – but after the first session that went and he's always so keen to come now. We travel 50 miles each way every two weeks and don't begrudge a centimetre of it. I pick him up tired and grumpy from school and he sits silent in the car munching his sandwiches on the way. On the way back he's transformed – bright, perky and communicative. We turn off the music and talk.'

Parent of nine-year-old boy with complex heart conditions with several in-patient admissions
'It is very beneficial for him to meet other cardiac children outside the ward.'
'There are times when P. feels very much alone, and it is beneficial for him to meet and play with other children who struggle with the same or similar difficulties as he does.'
'Over recent months he is more comfortable and confident in his own skin. The Cardiac Art Therapy Group has been the consistent driving force in this shift for my son.'

Comment from a ten-year-old child attending the group
'I thought I was the only one.'

First referrals were all children with arrhythmias,[1] but as the work progressed, criteria were broadened to include other heart conditions, as other cardiology consultants began to refer patients. Visual images produced in art therapy sessions were powerful, communicating the children's inner worlds without flinching (May 1975). The cardiology consultant suggested the work should be shown to a wider audience. Over time, there were five exhibitions, held in hospital settings and a gallery within Glasgow University. The work was professionally curated, mounted and presented, and was a source of pride and achievement to the children and their families.

The Senior Cardiac Nurses who were co-therapists in the groups were highly skilled nursing practitioners, whom had known many of the children over a long period of time and several of them from birth. This familiarity allowed them to move easily between joining in with the art-making to responding to the children's worries and medical queries as they arose. Some children carried defibrillators, a device which would restart their heart if it stopped. In early sessions, there were several defibrillators lined up on a shelf at the back of the art therapy space, and I was relieved to have medically trained staff present. Nurse co-therapists also became skilled in reading images. A nurse noticed that a mask painted with red and blue streams bore a strong resemblance to vascular blood flow; a painting done by a teenage boy directly after a heart check-up had within its abstract patterns shapes that closely resembled his heart trace. Their medical knowledge alerted them to communications I would have missed. Susan Bach (1966, 1975, 1990) is known for her extensive research into artwork by seriously ill children, believing that these were spontaneous depictions of symptoms and prognosis.

The group

In the group sessions, several children made images based on the TV programme 'Dr Who', the Time Lord who regenerates many times in a new form, as if conquering death. Many of these children had in-dwelling devices, pacemakers to control their heart rhythm. Monsters, such as bears, yeti, werewolves and ghosts were frequent themes. Malchiodi (1999) describes the appearance of monsters in drawings of young children affected by illness, seeing this as the illness perceived as external threat in monstrous form. Monsters are fellow travellers with humans, lurking in shadows at the edge of the path and the margins of society (Weegmann, 2008). A ten-year-old girl with an arrhythmia made a large colourful drawing of her family. Just as I thought she had finished she added a ghost and a question mark. Both she and her father had been diagnosed with arrhythmias following his collapse. Malchiodi (1999) describes ghosts as spiritual aspects, perceptions and experiences beyond the self.

Many children were lonely, and often excluded from play at other children's homes due to the adults' anxiety around their heart condition. Some had experienced verbal and occasionally physical bullying. The consultant had told me that children with heart conditions often had anger issues, however, while they were wary of others, clearly longed for social contact and friendship. Most children joined the groups after a few one-to-one sessions; a few highly anxious children remained in individual sessions for months. Apart from one teenage boy who asked to attend with his siblings, all children joined the groups. Two children died over the course of the group.

Case study

Charlie was nine years old when first referred to the Art Therapy Clinic. He had an arrhythmia and was frequently excluded from school for angry outbursts resulting in violence towards teaching staff and other children. He also had a diagnosis of ADHD. Charlie had been removed from his family of origin at the age of two, after experiencing physical cruelty and severe neglect. He had been fostered since then with a very experienced foster mother who offered excellent care and a deep attachment to him. He attended the Cardiac Art Therapy Clinic for five years, in individual sessions for the first year followed by dyadic sessions with a boy the same age the following year, with them both joining the group together. Charlie took on the role of big brother to younger children in the groups. He was used to caring for foster siblings, often babies, and was remarkably patient with his group 'siblings'. He was now in High School, in top academic groups in all subjects. In early group sessions, Charlie was impulsive. In one session, he dropped a balloon filled with paint on a large drawing he had made of a boy, a huge explosion which obliterated the drawing and splattered the whole room. In another session, Charlie poured PVA glue down the sink, blocking the drain and necessitating a plumber dismantling the whole sink and issuing a warning to the group not to repeat this

(a) (b)

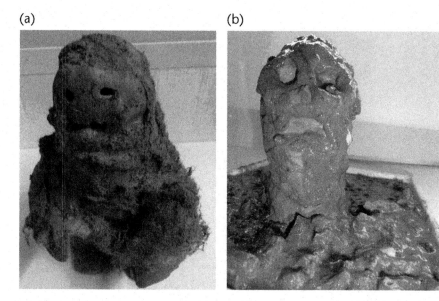

FIGURE 9.6 Monsters, clay and paint

experiment. Gradually Charlie gained confidence in his creative abilities, making a castle from a cardboard box with two turrets for guards. His foster mother noticed that the hospital incinerator chimney outside the window had the same shape as Charlie's castle turrets. This conversation showed me that parents were beginning to pay more attention to the children's art images, seeing them as important communications of feelings and responses to the world. Charlie was frightened of lifts; the art therapy room was on the sixth floor. He ran all the way up the stairs, and I would hear his running footsteps along the corridor. In the early individual sessions, Charlie had made a clay cave, with a little clay cave baby with outstretched arms, as if wanting held. This piece was given central place in the exhibition. He and his dyadic companion, now a close friend, painted the art equipment, clay tools, scissors and brushes with gold paint, transforming them into precious objects, golden tools.

The child psychiatrist's perspective: art therapy for children at Yorkhill

In 1996, I was appointed as a consultant child psychiatrist at the Glasgow Children's Hospital, combining tasks in the Child Psychiatry Ward with a leadership role for the development of the small liaison psychiatry service providing care for children in the hospital. The ward had been the physical base of the entire child psychiatry service but most psychiatric services were moving into new community-based mental health clinics. The ward was remaining on the hospital site. The in-patient service based in the ward was beginning to face challenges arising from the pending closure of most of the other similar units in Scotland.

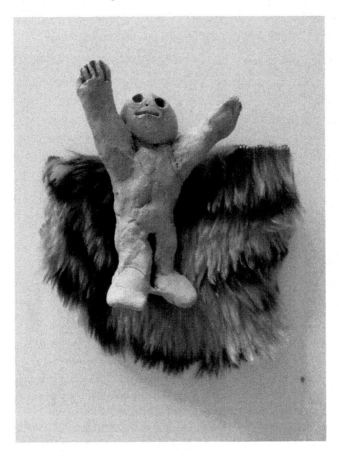

FIGURE 9.7 Cave baby

As a trainee in Manchester, I had been privileged to work as a co-therapist in a group alongside an art therapist and had observed the power of a non-directive art therapeutic approach with young people who were not responsive to talking therapies. As an undergraduate I had spent a year out of medicine, studying art history as an intercalated degree. These experiences contributed to my personal development and in my new post, I was open to less usual approaches to meeting challenges. The child psychiatry ward team had a small budget for creative therapists' time. Some staff had great skills in various therapeutic modalities, but the core team did not include the skill-set of art therapy. The small liaison team comprised sessions from a consultant colleague and an experienced charge nurse, supported by other staff in an ad hoc fashion. There was also a strong department of clinical psychology in the hospital with an emphasis on early intervention. In the paediatric departments of the hospital there were play specialists but no formal non-verbal psychotherapeutic work beyond traditional uses of play and drawing in clinical interventions.

In time, with supportive management, it was possible to negotiate the development of the in-patient child psychiatry ward as a regional resource. Funding for creative therapy input to the ward was consolidated to allow the establishment of a long-term commitment to purchasing therapist time and the Senior OT led to the development of a group programme with a weekly art therapy group as the core non-directive component. Individual art therapy sessions for ward patients were a later development following the team's recognition of the value of the modality.

In 2005, in somewhat more challenging conditions, the ward was established by NHS Scotland's National Services Division as National Child Psychiatry In-patient Unit. This led to further staffing developments, but the national commissioning process did not allow for the continuation of a joint service of in-patient and liaison psychiatry. The liaison team developed separately from the ward from this point, but I continued working with both teams.

With little evidence from UK paediatric practice to establish a case, there was no way to achieve an art therapy service for children in the paediatric wards of the hospital at the time of service development for the ward. The developing service focussed on making strong relationships with paediatric staff to support best practice in identifying mental health need and managing this with the resources in the hospital, making best use of the existing skills. This style of working did not necessarily lead to individual referrals and we developed a system of recording consultations in files with no identifying details relating to the patient or patients discussed. Thus, psychiatric expertise could contribute to children's care without formal referral and creation of a mental health record. Children were seen in the wards or sometimes jointly with paediatric staff in clinics and the scope for longer-term therapeutic work was limited. This liaison approach required the development of skills in neuropsychiatry and biological aspects of the interplay of mental disorder and paediatric practice. The insights into the impact of anxiety in health settings found in the work of Donald Winnicott (1965) and Isobel Menzies Lyth (1960, 1988) were also a guide to our collaboration with paediatric colleagues.

Adrian Sutton, one of my trainers in Manchester, has written of the interplay of paediatric and psychiatric services and the positive impacts upon development that may come from constructive contact with paediatric teams (Sutton, 2013). Chronic disorder brings a range of influences to play in the development of the sick child. Whilst it is well recognised that chronic childhood illness may lead to an increased risk of psychiatric disorder, there is less written about gains that may flow from successful adjustment to childhood illness (Gledhill et al., 2000). My own research with young people who had grown up with end-stage renal failure suggested that although illness is an adversity there maybe benefits arising through adjustment (Reynolds et al., 1993). Children attending a well-run paediatric service may also benefit from health education in relation to attitudes to alcohol, drugs, diet and exercise. Sadly, a small number of children may experience a consistency of care from hospital staff that is not available in other areas of their life. Paediatric staff, aware of their role in supporting children and families in adjustment to illness through key stages of development, may improve other outcomes in addition to dealing with the challenges of chronic disease.

Both paediatrics and child psychiatry have been influenced by the work of Winnicott and the notion of a developmental line through play to creativity. I found that Winnicott's (1980) account of 'the Piggle' provided a way of encouraging a different perspective on the therapeutic opportunities in a doctor's relationship with a child. Medical training involves learning to observe outward signs of health and disease. In paediatrics, this includes both pattern recognition in the diagnosis of congenital conditions and observing unspoken intra-familial communications in the clinic. Play is sometimes used in support of paediatric assessments and interventions but its value in communication with children can be overlooked. In supervision, trainees could reflect on the value of attending to non-verbal communication. This could involve monitoring family and individual behaviour and non-verbal communication through play or other creative activities available in a paediatric clinic. Paediatric doctors and nurses are careful observers of children's behaviour, play and their creativity. Based upon my own experiences in training, I suggested that young paediatricians use simple art materials (paper and coloured pencils) to enhance communication. I encouraged the use of the squiggle game (Winnicott, 1974) as a way of opening up shared non-verbal play in the absence of toys and when children were resistant to communicating by other means.

As the liaison service developed, it became possible to offer more therapeutic work with children. In supervision of weekly non-directive therapy, it was a pleasure to see the added value that long-term individual work with children brought to the service, bringing practitioners to a more intensive involvement with children's worlds. Work in a hospital setting is often limited by practical constraints, such as the lack of space to store toys and children's work. Two-dimensional creativity on paper was often the most manageable option in our setting. The need for an art therapist's eye in the liaison service became more apparent as the team developed.

Glasgow child psychiatry became integrated with adolescent psychiatry in community Child and Adolescent Mental Health Services (CAMHS). This co-incided with an increase in psychiatric prescribing for young people and increased awareness of the risk of cardiac arrhythmias, a dangerous side effect caused by some psychiatric medications. The need for better links with cardiology services lead to my spending more time in discussion with Dr Karen McLeod, the Consultant Cardiologist, a specialist in disorders of heart rhythm. Karen spoke about the level of mental health need amongst her patients, for some of whom the onset of palpitations might be a warning of the possibility of sudden death. Some patients had familial disorders diagnosed before they developed symptoms as a result of screening following the collapse or even death of a family member. Karen was aware that for some families, the verbal exploration of feelings in traditional models of mental health services did not suit their needs. She wondered if certain cardiac conditions create a particular kind of anxiety in the family, and in the child, 'a fear for which there are no words'.

Discussion with Karen articulated a key issue in liaison psychiatry. It is normally the business of psychiatrists to help their patients and those around them face and deal with reality but where sudden death is a high risk the task may change. Some realities can be overwhelming, and the therapeutic task can only proceed at a pace tolerable for those involved. It had been most unusual for the cardiac team to refer patients to liaison psychiatry and I had only been able to speculate about the reason for this. Karen told me about referrals to the clinical psychology service where patients often did not persevere with contact. It seemed to us both that the task of putting anxiety into words was too much for the families of some children.

Although the heart is seen in medical history as seat of emotions (Stolberg, 2019), there is limited engagement with psychological medicine in cardiology practice, even in adults where the prognostic importance of mental disorder in IHD is well known (Pedersen and Andersen, 2018). The psychological literature relating to children with heart disease is relatively sparse and it is not possible to define an adequate evidence base to discuss the specific challenges of chronic cardiac conditions in childhood.

Speaking with Karen about her patients I was thinking about work going on in the ward. As art therapist, Sheena worked at the pace set by the patient, images emerged and words followed when the time was right. My thoughts turned to the possibility that art therapy might be helpful for cardiac patients. Sheena had treated one of Karen's patients in a different setting and all concerned had felt was very helpful. It seemed that a three-way conversation could be useful. After reflection, we decided to find a way to set up a pilot project at the children's hospital. Our aim was to explore the potential of art therapy in adjustment to illness. Initially, we would focus on Karen's patients with familial arrhythmias.

The plan to offer an intervention to children with life-limiting illness needed to be progressed with due care to ensure that any negative consequences would be minimised. Central to this was the involvement of the cardiac nursing team. Cardiac nurses carry considerable knowledge of the family and social background of their patients. They are the first port of call for families seeking support with managing a cardiac condition and they bring their perspective into the decision-making process of the cardiac team. Two specialist cardiac nurses showed great interest in the plan to offer art therapy and were integral to the service development.

Any development had to fit with plans to improve mental health services in the hospital. Colleagues in psychiatry and clinical psychology had a positive view of art therapy. There was a consensus that a non-verbal therapeutic approach could be helpful for children who had not been able to use other approaches.

Cardiology support in the development of art therapy reflected the importance of the professional eye. The diagnostic power of visual observation is a distinguishing feature of the physician's gaze. Describing the development of the medical profession, Foucault (1976) wrote 'One must, as far as possible, make science ocular'. In 1926, a pioneer of medical education, Sir William Osler, wrote, 'Observe, record, tabulate, communicate' (Bean, 1950). Medical training still emphasises the development of observation. Cardiac conditions are frequently characterised by visual signs: from the reading of the electro-cardiograph to the blue extremities of peripheral circulatory failure and the dramatic sight of colour draining in syncope. The experience of learning to look and see is common to training in art history, art therapy and medicine. The observational skills of colleagues involved in the development of the art therapy group lead to rich conversations about the children's creative work and facilitated a therapeutic collaboration.

It was agreed that art therapy would not be a preventative strategy or a re-creational or diversional activity. The proposal was for an intervention that might be offered to some quite troubled children. It was accepted that any development of art therapy needed a governance framework but the approach to recruitment of patients should avoid formalities that might put off those in need of help. Thus, there was an agreement that patients would attend art therapy as part of paediatric treatment with no threshold of referral to CAMHS required. As it would clearly be inappropriate to record details of therapy in a hospital file, the art therapist would keep her own records according to the protocol of her agency but also produce a short report for the paediatric file. The children's work could be kept safely in a store-room in the liaison psychiatry base until therapy was completed, when work would be either returned to the child or destroyed when this not possible. Records of supervision would be held securely as liaison psychiatry 'consultation files'. This model of care provision depended upon trust between paediatric consultants who retained overall clinical responsibility for their patients' care, the psychiatric consultant (myself) supervising therapy and the service provider (Creative Therapies), who employed the art therapist (Sheena). The management of this complex arrangement required both the creative approach of the manager in the paediatric hospital, where ad hoc arrangements for 'add on' care were not uncommon, and an openness to collaboration from managers in CAMHS and Creative Therapies.

In the development of mental health services within general hospitals, mental health professionals must interact with colleagues within a health setting that has different values and priorities from those they experience in training in the community or in specialist mental health institutions. The concept of liaison psychiatry contains within it an acknowledgement of the accommodations necessary for mental health services to function within an acute hospital (Kraemer, 2010). Art therapy in a children's hospital offers particular opportunities and challenges (Wajcman, 2018).

The Glasgow children's hospital was an early adopter of the United Nations Convention on the Rights of the Child (1990), recognising the importance of play and creativity in a health setting. The built environment contains spaces reserved both for education and play, with many examples of the use of play and art materials on display. Nevertheless, the main tasks of the hospital may cut across boundaries that generally surround psychotherapeutic group work. The specific requirements of an art therapy group for a suitable space available at a regular time with reliable support for attendance of staff and patients can be understood as similar to those required in a hospital school classroom but the psychological boundaries around the space are different. Identification of the group as a therapeutic activity within the oversight of psychiatry provided a framework for practice that was already established in the hospital. The liaison team had a good relationship with other paediatric services sharing a disused ward space. None of these services had clinics on Friday afternoons, so the use of the shared waiting room for the group became a physical enactment of this containing framework.

Supervision included fortnightly meetings with Sheena and less frequent joint meetings with Sheena and members of the cardiology team. The content of Sheena's supervision included much that was familiar to me from other work supervising groups, but the striking difference was the fascination of seeing the unfolding development of form, colour and imagery in the work that was brought to sessions. The work varied from fine pencil drawings to shapeless lumps of clay but as the individual children, represented by their creations, grew in my mind I began to see the power of apparently unconscious expression through free access to art materials provided in the group.

As supervisor, I found that I was also a mediator between differing perspectives of art therapy. For the nurses involved, the group was an entirely new experience. Sheena's ability to tolerate children's destructive urges and apparently wasteful use of materials went against their training. For paediatric staff from other teams passing the art therapy room, the activities within were a source of fascination. There is always a danger that mental health services in acute hospitals are seen as alien, incomprehensible and even eccentric but the established reputation and relationships of the liaison team helped to place this new and colourful activity within a proper therapeutic context.

The idea of exhibiting artwork came from cardiology staff and was in keeping with the culture of the hospital. I found it hard to square this with my notions of the confidentiality of the therapeutic process but the reaction of those involved convinced me of the value a plan to exhibit the work. I was struck by the power of a child's colourful image of a fortress appearing on the hospitals' video screens advertising the first exhibition, by chance but most symbolically sited in a disused operating theatre of our neighbouring adult infirmary. Attending the exhibition, seeing the work together with the children, their families and professionals, confirmed the importance of this departure from my pre-conceived ideas of the need for a closed setting for therapy.

In order to explore the impact of the intervention, we sought to examine numeric data. During initial evaluation of the clinic, an attempt was made to use the Strengths and Difficulties Questionnaire (SDQ) – a questionnaire measure of psychopathology widely used in CAMHS (Vostanis, 2006). The SDQ was offered to children and parents after their second attendance and again after attendance for a period (of variable duration ten weeks to three years). Working without a receptionist or clinic administrator, it was hard to achieve the desired rate of response from both child and parent. Sixteen children were subjects of at least one valid questionnaire and seven of these had high or very high scores for total difficulties, with 'very high' impact of symptoms in six cases (equivalent to the 'most troubled' 5% of a population sample). 'High or very high' scores are indicators of levels of psychopathology that might lead to CAMHS referral. These scores suggest that the clinic was attracting a mixture of referrals, some with significant overt mental health disorder and others who were not symptomatic to such a degree. Findings from nine children where parental SDQs had been returned on more than one occasion (at the start of treatment and after participating in therapy) indicated a possible trend towards improvement but there were insufficient responses for meaningful analysis. The young peoples' own reports in eight cases with two valid questionnaires showed a sense of improvement overall but numbers were insufficient for formal analysis.

In addition to questions about symptoms, young people and parents were asked at follow up if the group was 'helpful' in other ways. The response was scored from 0 to 3 with 0 being 'not at all' and 3 being 'a great deal'. Parents responded in seven cases with a positive mean score of 2. Young people gave a response in seven cases with a mean score of 1.9. No one described the group as 'not helpful'. The feedback was that group was seen positively by both young people and parents both in relation to young people dealing with their difficulties and also in less specific ways (about which one can speculate taking account of other comments, e.g. that it was good to meet others with similar difficulties). Taken together with the measurements of change described by the young people, the overall finding is positive.

Despite considerable support within the hospital, resources did not allow for a continuation of this approach to evaluation. With no research assistant, receptionist or administrator, the task of distributing and ensuring return of questionnaires proved incompatible with the engaging and relaxed arrangements for arrival and departure within the structure of the group. The importance of continuing to seek feedback from children, families and staff was recognised and actively pursued. In particular, it was helpful to have responses to questions put to key staff in cardiology.

The consultant paediatric cardiologist's feedback

My recollection is that Sheena and Michael came to ask me whether I thought art therapy might benefit other children with cardiac conditions, as I had seen such an extraordinary benefit in Mandy. I immediately thought of the children who have inherited rhythm conditions that can cause sudden death in them or members of their family. Indeed, some of the children had lost loved ones to the conditions. I could see how they were struggling to come to terms both with their loss and the realisation that they themselves may be at risk of dying suddenly. We decided to start art therapy with this particular group of children. We approached the Association for Children with Heart Disorders, asking for funding. They supported the art therapy servicefor two to three years, after which, because of its success, it was funded by the hospital. Art therapy proved to be so helpful that it was opened to children with other cardiac conditions.

Mandy was the first and at that time the only (as far as I was aware) patient of mine that had been to art therapy. It made such a difference to Mandy and I think has been instrumental in her recovery from a condition we thought to be terminal. Initially, there was mirth and scepticism, within the cardiology team, as there were to my previous attempts at persuading management to agree to funding a psychologist post for cardiology but in time, the attitudes changed to appreciating the value of psychological support including art therapy.

Initially, we focussed on patients with inherited cardiac rhythm disorders, but ultimately offered art therapy to any child with a heart condition, whom we thought might benefit.

The children's art images were so varied. Some were moving but some were quite shocking. The exhibitions were fantastic, and I was really proud of the work done, including how the children collaborated and supported each other. It was lovely to see how the children transformed and gained confidence over the weeks of art therapy.

Conclusion

Research in art therapy is at an early stage. In our hospital setting, an attempt was made to explore various methods of evaluating the clinical impact of the intervention. This project highlighted the importance of seeking feedback and reflecting upon outcomes, opening the work of art therapy to the observations of those less familiar with the discipline. Working with children with heart conditions strengthened our already-firm belief in the power of creativity as a force for healing and positive change. As anxiety lessened in the children, their ability to find the necessary visual symbols to contain primitive fears emerged. These symbols were highly individual, as each child found the capacity to work with personal metaphorical language to confront existential fears. To be able to adequately support authentic expression of individual lived experience, the art therapist needed the cultural knowledge to recognise the symbols as they appeared. The art therapy room with its rich variety of well-maintained art materials provided the tools and armour. Part of the therapist's role is as keeper of the artwork, ensuring it is safely stored over the course of therapy. Both children represented had long engagements with art therapy over a period of years. The permanent nature of art images allows them to be revisited in a series of ritualistic transactions between the therapist and client. Primitive fears were safely contained. Words felt inadequate and overwhelming, but the meaning was acknowledged in the symbolised image. Images work on many levels, holding ambiguity, containing paradox, which is often at the heart of therapy of any depth.

With acknowledgements to Jamie Redfern, Sr Eileen Fern and our colleagues at the Glasgow Children's Hospital. With thanks to the Glasgow Children's Hospital Charity and the Scottish Association for Children with Heart Disorders.

Note

1 A cardiac arrhythmia is the medical term for an irregular heartbeat or abnormal heart rhythm.

References

Aldridge, F. (1998) 'Chocolate or shit: Aesthetics and cultural poverty in art therapy with children', *Inscape,* 3, pp. 2–9.

Appleton, V.E. (1993) 'An art therapy protocol for the medical trauma setting', *Art Therapy: Journal of American Art Therapy Association,* 10(2), pp. 71–77.

Bach, S. (1966) *Life paints its own span: On the significance of spontaneous pictures by severely Ill children.* Zurich: Susan-Bach-Stiftung and Daimon Verlag.

Bean, W.B. (ed.) (1950) *Sir William Osler Aphorisms collected by RB Bean.* New York: Henry Schumann Inc.

Bettelheim, B. (1976) *The uses of enchantment: The meaning and importance of fairy tales.* London: Penguin Books.

Bion, W.R. (1962a, 1977) *Learning from experience, seven servants.* New York: Aranson.

Bion, W.R. (1962b, 1967) *A theory of thinking, second thoughts.* New York: Aranson, pp. 110–119, 1967.

Bion, W.R. (1964) *Container and contained. Elements of psychoanalysis.* London: Heinemann.

Bion, W.R. (1990) *Brazilian lectures: 1973.* 1st edn. Sao Paulo: Routledge.

Birtchnell, J. (1984) 'Art as a form of psychotherapy' in Dalley, T. (ed.) *An introduction to the use of art as a therapeutic technique.* London: Tavistock Publications.

Bissonnet, J. (2015) 'Intimations of mortality: art therapy with children and young people with life-threatening or life-limiting illnesses' in Liebmann, M., and Weston, S. (eds.) *Art therapy and physical conditions.* London: Jessica Kingsley.

Bradley, C. (1999) 'Making sense of symbolic communication', in Hardwick, A., and Woodhead, J. (eds.) *Loving, hating and survival.* London: Ashgate Publishing.

Brown, Lawrence J. (2012) 'Bion's discovery of alpha function: Thinking under fire on the battlefield and in the consulting room', *International Journal of Psychoanalysis,* 5, p. 93.

Caffo, E., and Belaise, C. (2003) 'Psychological aspects of traumatic injury in children and adolescents', *Child and Adolescent Psychiatric Clinics of North America,* 12(3), pp. 493–535.

Case, C., and Dalley, T. (eds.) (1999) *Working with children in art therapy.* 4th edn. London: Routledge.

Case, C., and Dalley, T. (2006) *The handbook of art therapy.* 2nd edn. London: Routledge, pp. 89-112.

Casement, P.J. (1985) *On learning from the patient.* London: Tavistock Publications.

Councill, T. (1999) 'Art therapy with pediatric cancer patients', in Malchiodi, C. (ed.), *Medical art therapy with children.* London: Jessica Kingsley.

Dalley, T. (2006) *Theoretical developments and influences on current art therapy practice. In The Handbook of Art Therapy,* Hove and New York: Routledge.

Fischer, M. (2015) 'War zones: art therapy with an eleven-year-old boy with Crohn's disease' in Liebmann, M., and Weston, S. (eds.) *Art therapy with physical conditions.* London: Jessica Kingsley.

Franks, M., and Whitaker, R. (2007) The image, mentalisation and group art psychotherapy. *International Journal of Art Therapy,* June 12(1), p. 2.

Foucault, M. (1976) *The birth of the clinic.* London: Tavistock, pp. 88–91.

Furth, G. (1988) *The secret world of drawings: A Jungian approach to healing through art.* Toronto: Inner City Books.

Gledhill, J., Rangel, L.M., and Garralda, E.M. (2000) 'Surviving chronic physical illness: psychosocial outcome in adult life', *Archives of Disease in Childhood,* 83, pp. 104–110.

Gunter, M. (2000) 'Art therapy as an intervention to stabilize the defences of children undergoing bone marrow transplantation', *Arts Psychotherapy,* 27(1), pp. 3–14.

Heidegger, M. (1962) *Being and time.* Oxford: Blackwell Publishing.

Jung, C.G. (1953) *Collected works, Volume 12: Psychology and alchemy.* Bollingen: Pantheon.

Killick, K. (2000) 'The art room as container in analytical art psychotherapy with patients in psychotic states', in Gilroy, A., and McNeilly, G. (eds.) *The changing shape of art therapy: New developments in theory and practice.* London: Jessica Kingsley.

Kramer, E. (2000) *Art as therapy: Collected papers.* London: Jessica Kingsley.

Kraemer, S. (2010) 'Liaison and co-operation between paediatrics and mental health', *Paediatrics and Child Health,* 20(8), pp. 382–387.

Kris, E. (1953) *Psychoanalytic explorations in art.* London: Allen & Unwin.

La Nave, F. (2015) 'Theatre of the image and group interaction', in Waller, D. (ed.) *Group interactive art therapy.* London: Routledge.

Laing, J. (1974) 'Art therapy: Painting out the puzzle of the inner mind', *New Psychiatry,* 6(28 Nov), pp. 16–18

Lowenfeld, V. (1957) *Creative and mental growth.* 3rd edn. New York: The MacMillan Company.

Malchiodi, C. (ed.) (1999) 'Understanding somatic and spiritual aspects of children's art expressions', *Medical art therapy with children.* London: Jessica Kingsley. 173-196.

May, R. (1994) *The courage to create.* New York and London: W.W.Norton & Company.

Menzies Lyth, I. (1960) 'A case-study in the functioning of social systems as a defence against anxiety. A report on a study of the nursing service of a general hospital', *Human Relations,* 13(2), pp. 95–121.

Menzies Lyth, I. (ed.) (1988) 'Staff support systems: Task and anti-task in adolescent institutions', *Containing anxiety in institutions: Selected essays* (Vol. 1). London: Free Association Books. 222-235.

Miller, C. (2016) *Arts therapists in multidisciplinary settings: Working together for better outcomes.* London: Jessica Kingsley.

O'Brien, F. (2004) 'The making of mess in art therapy', *Inscape,* 9(1), pp. 2–12.

Ogden, T.H. (2004) On holding and containing, being and dreaming. *International Journal of Psychoanalysis,* 85(6), pp. 1349–1364.

Pedersen, S.S., and Andersen, C.M. (2018) 'Minding the heart: Why are we still not closer to treating depression and anxiety in clinical cardiology practice?' *European Journal of Preventive Cardiology,* 25(3), pp. 244–246.

Prokofiev, F. (1998) 'Adapting the art therapy group for children', in Skaife, S., and Huet, V. (eds.) *Art psychotherapy groups: Between pictures and words.* London: Routledge.

Reynolds, J.M., Morton, M.J.S., Garralda, M.E., Postlethwaite, R.J., and Goh, D. (1993) 'Psychosocial adjustment of adult survivors of a paediatric dialysis and transplantation programme', *Archives of Disease in Childhood,* 68, pp. 104–110.

Shore, A. (2013) *The practitioner's guide to child art therapy: Fostering creativity and relational growth*. UK and New York: Routledge.

Simpson, C. (2015) 'The power of the image in memory-making with children with life-limiting conditions', in Liebman, M., and Weston, S. (eds.) *Art therapy with physical conditions*. London: Jessica Kingsley.

Stolberg, M. (2019) 'Emotions and the body in early modern medicine', *Emotion Review*, 11(2), pp. 113–122.

Sutton, A. (2013) *Paediatrics, psychiatry and psychoanalysis*. UK and New York: Routledge.

Tjasink, M. (2010) 'Art psychotherapy in medical oncology: A search for meaning', *International Journal of Art Therapy*, 15, p. 2.

United Nations Convention on Rights of the Child. (1989) New York: United Nations General Assembly, Resolution 44/25 20 November 1989.

Vostanis, P. (2006) 'Strengths and difficulties questionnaire: Research and clinical applications', *Current Opinion in Psychiatry*, 19(4), pp. 367–372.

Wajcman, K. (2018) 'Developing an art therapy program in a children's hospital', *Art Therapy*, 35(2), pp. 104–107.

Weegmann, M. (2008) 'Monsters: the social-unconscious life of 'others' and a note on the origins of group therapy', *Group Analysis,* 41(3), 291–300. doi: 10.1177/0533316408094904

Winnicott, D.W. (1958) *Collected Papers: through paediatrics to psycho-analysis*. USA: Basic Books.

Winnicott, D.W. (1964) *The child, the family, and the outside world*. London: Penguin.

Winnicott, D.W. (1965) *Maturational processes and the facilitating environment*. London: Hogarth Press and the Institute of Psychoanalysis.

Winnicott, D.W. (1974) *Playing and reality*. London: Penguin.

Winnicott, D.W. (1980). *The piggle*. London: Penguin.

Wood, M. (1984) 'The child and art therapy', in Dalley, T. (ed.) *Art as therapy*. London and New York: Tavistock/Routledge.

The World Health Organization (2010) *Framework for action on inter-professional education and collaborative practice*. Geneva: World Health Organization.

Yalom, I.D. (1980) *Existential psychotherapy*. New York: Basic Books.

Yalom, I.D. (1998) *The Yalom reader*. 1st edn. New York: Basic Books.

INDEX